What people are saying about The Perricone Weight-Loss Diet

66 I'm eighteen days into the Perricone weight-loss program and the rewards continue to keep me moving forward. I have lost eight pounds, much to my delight! My skin looks great and the most amazing result has been my vitality. I usually feel fatigue every day. I never feel tired anymore. I sleep through the night, which is amazing, and wake up feeling refreshed. Oh, and I'm not all puffy when I wake up. Love that! 99

—LUCILLE JACCARINO

66 I have just loved my whole Perricone experience. I have been on the program nineteen days and have lost nine pounds. I feel very positive about this diet—and I managed to stay on the diet with no problems while keeping up with my studies at Harvard Law School. My skin looks so much better than it ever has. I have never been able to go out without tons of foundation on and now I wear none. I never expected to enjoy 'dieting' so much. I have continued with the diet and have lost about three more pounds. I have nothing but the highest regards for this program and can't stop talking about it to everyone I know. 99

—JEANINE ZALDUENDO

66 I've suffered with head and stomach problems since high school. During the last ten years, the migraines were more frequent and pronounced. Symptoms included but were not limited to sensitivity to light and sound, nausea, and vomiting. As an adult, I *always* got a migraine with the start of my menstrual cycle, except this past month. If you look in my journal, I marked a few days as PMS (craving days) and MC (menstrual cycle) days. However, I didn't mention headache because I never had one. Equally important, is that I didn't suffer from stomach problems. I won't gross you out with the details, let's just say, not once did I double over from stomach spasms. "In fact, during the Perricone diet I didn't have a migraine or stomach spasm. This opportunity was not a diet for me but a life-changing experience. The Perricone diet is how I plan to eat for the rest of my life. 99

—EVANGELINE COSTA

66 I was very pleased with this program! I was able to lose nine pounds and not miss a beat pursuing my architecture degree at Columbia! I have been very vocal about the diet to my friends and some of my mother's older friends because it was such a positive experience. 99

—Ashley Simone

66 Great results with the Perricone diet—sixteen pounds in four weeks! 99

—David Keyt

66 I am so excited to have lost twelve pounds—just in time for my wedding. And I really enjoyed this diet! Since the conclusion of the Perricone diet, I have managed to keep the twelve pounds off by eating in moderation. I have lost two additional pounds and am currently trying to maintain this new lifestyle and new body! Although I cannot stay away from all of the bad carbs completely, I feel the diet gave my body and metabolism a kick start. In addition, I am now aware of what certain foods can do to my body and how I feel after eating things like bread, red meat, and sweets. Almost three months later, I find I will need to do a huge alteration on my wedding dress around the chest, waist, and hip area. It is making my wedding plans all the more exciting and I am actually looking forward to my next fitting! I hope I continue with this lifestyle and thank Dr. Perricone tremendously for giving me the opportunity! 99

—Coleen Aldanese

66 I feel great and am amazed at such dramatic results. I lost sixteen pounds while enjoying three meals and two snacks per day! It has been thirty-eight days since the program formally concluded and I resolved to stay on a modified version of Dr. Perricone's diet. This week was a breakthrough. I'm now down more than twenty pounds (ten percent of my body weight) and am at the weight I was when our first child (who is now seventeen) was born. I've added more healthy snacks now and slightly larger meal portions. I have no desire for red meat or processed foods and I feel fantastic!
"My wife, Carol, and I have recommended the program to many of our friends and co-workers because we believe so strongly in the philosophy behind it. 99

—Jay Scheiner

66 After losing fifteen pounds you can bet that I am a strong advocate
of the Perricone Weight-Loss Diet! 99
—Barbara Clarke-Ruiz

66 I loved the Perricone Weight-Loss Diet–I lost ten pounds!
It was so perfect. 99
—Juliana Pereira

66 I lost ten pounds in the first ten days and *never* went hungry. 99
—Eric Blinderman

Also by Nicholas Perricone, M.D.

The Wrinkle Cure
The Perricone Prescription
The Perricone Prescription Personal Journal
The Acne Prescription
The Clear Skin Prescription
The Perricone Promise

The Perricone Weight-Loss Diet

The Perricone Weight-Loss Diet

A Simple 3-Part Plan to Lose the Fat,
the Wrinkles, and the Years

Nicholas Perricone, M.D.

BALLANTINE BOOKS

NEW YORK

No book can replace the diagnostic expertise and medical advice of a trusted physician.
Please be certain to consult with your doctor before making any decisions that
affect your health, particularly if you suffer from any medical condition or
have any symptom that may require treatment.

Copyright © 2005 by Nicholas V. Perricone, M.D.

Published in the United States by Ballantine Books,
an imprint of The Random House Publishing Group,
a division of Random House, Inc., New York.

BALLANTINE and colophon are registered
trademarks of Random House, Inc.

LIBRARY OF CONGRESS CATALOGING-IN-PUBLICATION DATA

Perricone, Nicholas.
The Perricone weight-loss diet : a simple 3-part plan to lose the fat, the wrinkles,
and the years / by Nicholas Perricone– 1st ed.
p. cm.
Includes bibliographical references and index.
ISBN 0-345-48593-9 (alk. paper)
1. Reducing diets.   2. Weight loss.   3. Nutrition.   I. Title.
RM222.2.P4346 2005
613.2'5–dc22   2005048327

Printed in the United States of America on acid-free paper

www.ballantinebooks.com

24687531

FIRST EDITION

Book design by Michaelis/Carpelis Design Associates Inc.

Acknowledgments

Anne Sellaro again leads these acknowledgments as friend, colleague, collaborator, agent, and all-around ally. Her matchless skills, creativity, enthusiasm, and tireless support enable me to bring my message to millions of people worldwide.

I would also like to thank all of my many friends and colleagues including:

Caroline Sutton, Gina Centrello, Libby McGuire, Anthony Ziccardi, Tom Perry, Kim Hovey, Rachel Bernstein, Cindy Murray, Brian Mclendon, Lisa Barnes, and the entire team at Random House including their outstanding sales force.

David Vigliano and Elise Petrini at Vigliano Associates

Tony Tiano, Lennlee Keep, Eli Brown, and team at Santa Fe Productions

The Public Broadcasting Service (PBS-TV)

Harry Preuss, M.D., F.A.C.N.

Michigan State University College of Human Medicine

Edward Magnotti

Ed Hookstratten

Sharyn Kolberg

Craig Weatherby

Ed and Elizabeth Walsh

Richard Post

The team at N.V. Perricone M.D., Ltd.

Our retail partners Neiman Marcus, Nordstrom, Sephora, Saks, Henri Bendel's, Clyde's on Madison, Belk's, and Parisian

Senator and Mrs. Joseph Lieberman

My parents

My brother and sisters, Jimmy, Laura, June, and Barbara

My children, Jeffrey, Nicholas, and Caitie

Steve Mirabella, Sr.

Contents

Introduction

Writing *The Perricone Weight-Loss Diet* is the cumulative result of decades of research into the role of inflammation in aging and age-related diseases, including obesity. In many ways this is the most exciting and revolutionary book that I have written to date. Scientists are rapidly acknowledging the role of inflammation in many diseases and chronic conditions. However, I believe this will be the first book that will clearly demonstrate how this subclinical, microscopic, invisible inflammation is responsible for a great number of metabolic problems, resulting in accelerated aging, serious health threats, unwanted weight gain, and obesity.

If this was not bad enough news for adults, there is now alarming new evidence that this diet-related inflammation is also causing weight gain and obesity in young children and adolescents, resulting in diseases and conditions such as type 2 diabetes and metabolic syndrome (discussed in detail in Chapter 6), which normally do not manifest until much later in life.

The alarming epidemic of obesity in this country has led the National Institutes of Health and other leading health organizations to revise the food pyramid we all learned in school. Now, for example, they are recommending a significant increase in the amounts of fruits and vegetables we eat, a move I heartily endorse, because these foods (along with fish such as wild Alaskan salmon) are great sources of antioxidants, Nature's natural anti-inflammatories.

That is good news, because I believe that the solution to the ever-growing problem of trying to lose weight and remain healthy is as close as your next meal. My research has shown that the chief therapeutic intervention to prevent weight gain (regardless of age) is the anti-inflammatory diet. I have observed significant weight loss in thousands of individuals who follow the simple formula of avoiding foods that are pro-inflammatory and choosing in their place foods with anti-inflammatory properties. *The Perricone Weight-Loss Diet* will introduce you to these foods, forever dispelling confusion when you are in the supermarket or at a restaurant. You will now have a simple, foolproof plan for healthy eating that will accelerate weight loss and enable you to keep it off—for life.

What is of particular interest to me is the fact that the same foods (those with anti-inflammatory properties) that fight many diseases, aging, sagging skin, and wrinkling, also cause **significant weight loss**—and they are safe for everyone, children and adults alike. At the same time, the foods that accelerate aging and put us at risk for disease and the loss of cognitive abilities (the pro-inflammatory foods) also **cause** weight gain. These foods and beverages also interfere with the body's natural ability to metabolize foods properly, making it increasingly difficult to lose unwanted weight.

The Perricone Weight-Loss Diet anti-inflammatory regimen is unique because people who follow the program not only experience **significant loss of body fat** in a short period of time, they also display incredible radiance and a greater appearance of youthfulness. The majority of weight-loss programs result in the opposite effect, a haggard, dull, and somewhat drawn appearance to the face and body after weight loss.

Another wonderful benefit is this: the weight loss from this anti-inflammatory diet is one of *body fat* and not muscle. It is vitally important to maintain muscle mass, because muscle is "metabolically active" and **burns** more **calories** than other body tissue, even when you're not moving. The Perricone Weight-Loss Diet plan not only maintains lean body tissue (muscle) but actually increases muscle mass, allowing those on the program to retain a more youthful appearance, maintain strength, and keep the weight off!

The Perricone Weight-Loss Diet delivers visible results—quickly. In addition, our emphasis is always on the positive benefits, such as increased radiance to the skin, decreased pore size, decreased puffiness under the eyes, more glamorous definition and contour to the cheekbone and jawline, an increase in overall skin tone, an attractive, lithe, and well-muscled figure—and, of course, an impressive weight loss.

As we embark on the Perricone Weight-Loss Diet, I want to personally give each of you my promise that this program will work for you in both the short and the long term. It is not a diet, but a lifestyle. It includes natural, unadulterated foods; nutritional supplements that help metabolize fat, burn calories, and maintain muscle mass; and simple exercise recommendations that accelerate the loss of fat and the increase of muscle.

Cumulatively, each tier will result in a slim, supple body, more energy, greater brain power, a radiant, glowing complexion, and increased feelings of well-being for you and every member of your family.

The secret to this successful weight-loss plan is simple: follow an anti-inflammatory lifestyle. The cornerstone is the anti-inflammatory diet, which carefully **controls blood sugar** and **insulin levels** and therefore automatically decreases the incidence of hypertension, type 2 diabetes, obesity, the risk of heart disease, and metabolic syndrome.

This focus on microinflammation as a factor in aging and obesity is an entirely novel and original concept. And it works every time.

Nicholas Perricone, M.D.
Madison, Connecticut

PART I

The Inflammation–Fat Connection

Chapter 1

Getting Started

The best way to predict the future is to invent it.
—ALAN KAY, COMPUTER GENIUS/VISIONARY

In writing this book, I have discovered that the greatest gift I can give my readers is permission to eat healthy and delicious food. This might seem strange considering this book is about weight **loss,** because traditional concepts of weight loss are all about **not** eating—nevertheless, it is a fact.

Statistics regarding obesity and excess weight are alarming. The International Obesity Task Force, which is advising the European Union, had estimated in 2003 that about 200 million of the 350 million adults living in what is now the European Union may be overweight or obese. The U.S. Census Bureau's *Census 2000* stated that nearly two-thirds of adults in the United States were overweight, and 30.5 percent were obese.

However, a closer evaluation of the figures in the latest analysis indicated that may be an underestimate.

We Americans (children and adults) are more confused than ever about what constitutes a healthy diet. According to statistics from the National Institutes of Health, the prevalence of obesity in the United States has almost doubled since 1980.

And for good reason. For the past several decades, we have been bombarded with all kinds of misinformation about what we should and should not eat or drink. As soon as one scientific study hits the newswires, another one with equally convincing yet contradictory data springs up. From books to videos we are assailed with confusing and opposing points of view from all kinds of experts and pseudoexperts. Consequently, figuring out what to eat and what to avoid has become increasingly difficult.

The Perricone Weight-Loss Diet cuts through the confusion and provides a simple, foolproof eating plan that will improve your health, help to fight the signs of aging, help you to lose weight, and prevent new weight gain. It all begins with learning which foods make this possible and which foods defeat our purpose.

BUT FIRST, SOME HISTORY

Back in the 1960s, the then-young baby boomers began a dietary "back to the land" revolution in protest of the post–World War II introduction of processed foods. In typical backlash fashion, everything this generation embraced had to be "whole," "natural," "fresh," "unprocessed," and grown without pesticides and chemical fertilizers. This was the beginning of the health food movement, which is stronger and more powerful than ever, and finally after more than four decades, is becoming increasingly mainstream.

That was the good news. The bad news is that this was the last positive dietary trend we have seen. Ever since then, we have had one dangerous and poorly-thought-out plan after another. In addition, fast food has now become a ubiquitous part of our landscape. According to Eric Schlosser, author of *Fast Food Nation,* on any given day one out of four Americans has a meal from a fast-food restaurant.

The 1970s saw the introduction of the Atkins low-carbohydrate, high-protein diet. At first glance, the concept made sense; however, there were a number of serious and dangerous flaws (some since amended), among them an overabundance of saturated fats. The '90s reintroduced this craze, slightly modified.

Perhaps the worst dietary craze belongs to the 1980s, which heralded the age of the no-fat diet. Supermarket shelves were flooded with high-glycemic carbohydrate foods, offering little in the way of nutrients, but plenty in the way of empty calories. These foods became dietary mainstays for many people, especially women, who found themselves indulging in snack foods such as reduced-fat "baked" potato and corn chips, and fat-free rice and corn cakes, cookies, pretzels, and crackers. Suddenly millions of Americans were placing themselves in a chronic inflammatory condition. Why? Because eating these foods provokes a pro-inflammatory rapid rise in blood sugar, resulting in elevated insulin levels.

What Are High-Glycemic Foods?

According to the website www.glycemicindex.com, the "glycemic index is a ranking of carbohydrates based on their immediate effect on blood glucose (sugar) levels. It compares foods gram for gram of carbohydrates. Carbohydrates that break down quickly during digestion have the highest glycemic indexes. Carbohydrates that break down slowly, releasing glucose gradually into the bloodstream, have low glycemic indexes." There are numerous books and websites available that list glycemic values for all categories of food and beverages, including: www.glycemicindex.com. To prevent weight gain and/or lose the unwanted weight, we need to replace sugary and starchy foods and beverages with high-quality protein and low-glycemic fruits and vegetables, which have little effect on our blood sugar and insulin levels.

Insulin is an important hormone that helps the body utilize blood sugar for energy or store it as glycogen or fat. But if the insulin is released too quickly, it has a *pro-inflammatory* effect (explored further in Chapter 2). After a rapid rise, there will be a precipitous drop in blood sugar, resulting in feelings of hunger, which can lead to a vicious cycle of overeating. This is why a diet centered on breads, baked goods, snack foods, sweets, and other sugary, starchy foods results in unwanted weight gain and great difficulty in losing weight. Ironically, in this instance, it is not the caloric value of the foods causing the weight gain. In fact, a rice cake only has around 40 calories. However, because it is rapidly converted to sugar in the bloodstream, resulting in the insulin release, it will cause you to store body fat. An insulin release can result in the storage of body fat.

Our goal in the Perricone Weight-Loss Diet is to learn how to **recognize** and avoid sugary and starchy foods, so that we maintain even levels of blood sugar and insulin. Recognize? Yes, because many foods that look healthful can contain added sugars, dangerous trans fats (more about these later), and an ingredient called **high fructose corn syrup,** which will defeat weight-loss goals and have a negative impact on overall health. By following the Perricone Weight-Loss Diet, you will be able to control your appetite, prevent overeating, stop cravings, and burn excess fat for energy.

KEEPING IT SIMPLE

Some scientists and researchers believe that many of the health problems of today are caused by our departure from the hunter-gatherer diet, which consisted of nuts, seeds, berries, wild greens, roots, fruits, fish, fowl, and game. This is a fascinating theory and I do agree with the premise that natural, unprocessed foods are always the best choices. To be healthy and maintain normal weight we need all of the food groups— but not those that come from the laboratory. Our protein source needs to be pure, fresh (when possible) wild fish and other seafood, and free range chicken and turkey that are hormone and antibiotic free. Our carbohydrates need to be fresh fruits and vegetables, preferably organic. And we need good fats, such as those found in salmon, sardines, and other cold-water fish, extra virgin olive oil, nuts, seeds, avocado, and açaí (a Brazilian berry whose fatty-acid ratio resembles that of olive oil). These "good" fats will help us absorb nutrients from our vegetables and fruits, keep our cells supple, our skin glowing and wrinkle-free, our brains sharp, and our mood upbeat. We also need dietary fat to burn fat.

By upsetting the delicate balance with extreme fad diets and ridiculous concepts, whether it is no-carb or no-fat or whatever, we create ongoing physical and mental health problems, including obesity, accelerated aging, and wrinkling, sagging skin. It is no coincidence that the rise of antidepressants such as Prozac occurred during the nonfat food craze of the 1980s—after all, our brains are comprised mainly of fat, and when we starve our brains of valuable nutrients, we become depressed. Salmon, with its rich complement of essential fatty acids, has been shown to be an excellent treatment for depression. Some studies have shown that it is more effective than powerful drugs in treating depression—without the side effects (moderate regular exercise is also great for depression—especially when combined with the salmon-rich anti-inflammatory diet).

Our goal is to strive for balance and to use common sense when planning a meal.

Ava's transformation (see Ava's story on the following page) was, to say the least, impressive. If you follow the Perricone Weight-Loss Diet, you too can have impressive results.

But how does it all really work? The next several chapters will explain the science behind my revolutionary concepts and how you can make them work for you.

Ava's Story

One of the great joys of presenting my research at scientific conferences around the world is the opportunity to meet intriguing people from all walks of life. I first met Ava in Monaco, where I was delivering a keynote address at an international anti-aging conference. Ava was covering the conference for a major U.S.-based news weekly and approached me as I left the podium following my presentation.

"Excuse me, Dr. Perricone," she said. "I was fascinated by your talk and wonder if I might get a few quotes for my magazine." I was delighted to oblige, and we made plans to meet later at the Panorama Terrasse overlooking the spectacular Mediterranean.

After a delightful lunch, we were enjoying our aperitifs and the dazzling view of the sea from our cliffside terrace. "Dr. Perricone, I wonder if I might ask you for your professional advice," Ava asked rather timidly. As I nodded my acquiescence she began her story.

"I realize that your field of expertise is dermatology and anti-aging; however, during your lecture you mentioned something called the 'anti-inflammatory diet,' and how if one followed it, many of the conditions associated with aging, including unwanted weight gain, would be preventable. As I continued to listen to you, I realized that I have been doing EVERYTHING wrong in the diet and nutrition department. I started dieting in my twenties to lose an extra ten pounds. Over the years my weight has yo-yoed up and down until now at forty, I am saddled not only with the original ten pounds but another ten as well."

I asked Ava to outline a typical day's meal plan. "For breakfast I usually have a glass of orange juice, a cup of black coffee, and a toasted bagel with fat-free cream cheese. Lunch is usually a baked potato topped with nonfat sour cream. I like to snack on rice or corn cakes in the afternoon because they only have 40 calories each. For dinner I usually have a large salad with nonfat dressing and a skinless, boneless chicken breast. Truthfully, I am mystified by my difficulty in taking off weight because I NEVER eat fats or sweets of any kind," she added with a hint of desperation.

Ava's dilemma is not out of the ordinary. In fact, many of my female patients over the years have found themselves in the same difficult situation. In addition to the unwanted weight gain and great difficulty in taking off the weight, a diet centered on these types of foods accelerates the aging process and is highly damaging to the skin. I could see the protein deprivation in Ava's face; she looked exhausted and older than her years. I explained to Ava that she was committing three cardinal sins:

- failure to eat enough protein
- avoiding the good fats as well as the bad
- choosing carbohydrates that have a high-glycemic index, such as bagels, potatoes, and rice and corn cakes, in place of fresh fruits and vegetables

I outlined a simple regimen for Ava to follow consisting of three meals a day and two snacks. I also ▶

told her she needed to start taking three 1,000 mg capsules of high-quality fish oil three times per day for a total of nine per day, three packets per day with meals of a specially formulated weight management supplement containing all the nutrients she would need to facilitate weight loss. I promised to send her a list of recommended foods. She could mix and match her food choices from the list's quality protein sources, low-glycemic carbohydrates, and the right types of fats—with the basic admonition that she must include one of each of the food groups in every meal and snack. Also, to drink six to eight 8-ounce glasses of water per day.

Ava and I made plans to meet in New York a few weeks later; however, our busy schedules interfered and it wasn't until almost eight weeks later that we finally got together. As I entered the tea room I noticed a stunning brunette sitting at my favorite corner table. As I walked away to look for an empty table, I heard my name being called. "Dr. Perricone, over here." Imagine my surprise (and embarrassment) when I turned around and realized that I had walked right past Ava! The transformation was so dramatic that I had failed to recognize her. She was dressed in a stylish black wool suit with a form-fitting jacket that emphasized her beautiful figure and small waist. Her shoulder-length hair gleamed in the soft light of the tea room, while her beautiful skin glowed with the radiance of youth and health. Gone was the slightly overweight, harried and tired-looking journalist I had met in Monaco.

"Ava," I stammered, "you look fantastic!"

"Thank you, Dr. Perricone," she said. "Little did I know how fortuitous our first meeting would turn out to be. I quickly learned to love salmon, salads, and all of your recommended foods, because I noticed an immediate improvement in my skin, including a major decrease in puffiness. And I have so much more mental and physical energy!"

Ava had lost close to twenty pounds since our encounter in Monaco. It helped that she was very physically active thanks to the demands of her career, because exercise is critical to a successful weight-loss program. However, the key for Ava was reducing microinflammation by adding the right kind of fats to metabolize fat, while eliminating the wrong carbohydrates, which were causing her to store fat. The omega-3 fatty acids from fish oil capsules and plenty of seafood (especially the salmon) helped to rapidly facilitate her weight loss.

Later over dinner, Ava shared with me what had gone through her mind during my lecture. "I made up my mind that it was 'now or never.' I felt like you were tossing me a lifeline when you sent me that list of the right foods!" she confided.

As I sat contemplating her remarkable physical rejuvenation, I thought of the old proverb "Give a man a fish; you have fed him for today. Teach a man to fish, and you have fed him for a lifetime." Now that Ava had learned how to "fish" for the right foods, her problems with weight would forever be a thing of the past.

Chapter 2

The Inflammation–Aging– Disease–Obesity Connection

One's mind, once stretched by a new idea,
never regains its original dimensions.
— OLIVER WENDELL HOLMES

A s many readers of my earlier books know, the original anti-inflammatory diet is both a powerful antiaging, disease-fighting tool and the secret to clear, wrinkle-free skin. It was not specifically designed for weight loss. However, once I realized that people who needed to lose weight were rapidly losing it on this eating plan, I recognized a whole new world of potential for the overweight man or woman—whether he or she needed to shed a mere 10 pounds or was morbidly obese.

I altered and adapted the original anti-inflammatory diet to focus on the specific foods and supplements that were proven to accelerate healthy weight loss while maintaining muscle mass. In fact, the anti-inflammatory weight-loss diet in this book closely parallels the very diet that I follow on a daily basis. The recommended foods will not only enable you to quickly drop excess weight, you will find increased energy and an increased sense of mental well-being. When we realize that most dieters are subject to chronic crankiness, this is good news indeed.

In this book, you are going to learn some surprising facts—facts that actually startled the scientific community when they were first discovered. You are going to learn that excess body fat is a living, breathing, multiplying endocrine organ—and that fact alone ensures that the fatter you are, the fatter you will get. This book is going to change your ideas about weight gain and weight loss. It is not about your daily intake of fat—and it is not about cutting out the carbs. It is about something no other book has ever explained: the connection between inflammation and body fat (and the fact that one is never present without the other). You will learn what foods cause this inflammation, and how to decrease and prevent it, thereby permanently eliminating all weight problems.

INFLAMMATION 101

Let's take a look at what I mean by **inflammation.** Inflammation, which is the response of the body's immune system to infection or irritation, exists in a very wide spectrum. At the extreme end it causes visible redness and swelling, such as in sunburn or an injured finger. On the low end of the spectrum, the inflammation is invisible; we can't see it and we can't feel it. But it does exist, and it causes a host of health-related problems. The bright red and painful sunburn that exists at the extreme high end is usually present for only a short period of time. Physicians refer to this type of inflammation as "acute inflammation." The invisible inflammation that exists at the low end of the spectrum is usually present for longer periods of time and is termed "chronic inflammation."

The question you may be asking is, "If it is invisible, and we can't feel it, then how do we know that this low-grade inflammation exists?" The answer is simple: some of this inflammation *can* be detected under the microscope. However, low-grade inflammation can also be invisible even with a microscope because it exists on a molecular level, but it can be detected through chemical tests using special instruments.

Research indicates that the effects of this chronic, low-grade, invisible inflammation is at the basis of aging and age-related diseases such as cardiovascular disease, diabetes, certain forms of cancer, Parkinson's, Alzheimer's, and autoimmune diseases—and even wrinkled, sagging skin.

However, it doesn't stop there. I am now categorically stating that this same chronic, low-grade, invisible inflammation is at the very basis of excess body fat, out-of-control appetites, food cravings, food addictions, diabetes, and the inability to lose excess body weight.

If that is the case, you may be thinking, "Why don't I just go ahead and take an ibuprofen tablet and get thin?" Unfortunately, it is not that simple—especially when you consider this inflammation is not just a one-time event reacting to a one-time cause. Our bodies are under a constant barrage, a continual assault of physical insults resulting in this inflammation–beginning with that bag of potato chips and ending with the creation of a veritable factory in our body whose *one job* is to grow more fat cells and produce more inflammatory chemicals.

The answer lies in learning to recognize and avoid the factors that are creating the inflammation in the first place, and then, through natural means, reducing the existing inflammation to successfully lose the excess body fat. By embracing the anti-inflammatory diet and lifestyle, you will not only lose the weight, you will dramatically alter your quality of life–and increase your life expectancy.

The effect of this low-grade, invisible inflammation (also referred to as "subclinical" inflammation) has been at the cutting edge of medical science for the last decade, and it has been the focal point of my own research for the past two decades. After years of either being ignored or relegated to a "by-product" of the disease process, cellular inflammation is finally coming to the attention of the mainstream media, and in fact, was the topic of a cover story in *Time* magazine.

THE DANGERS OF INFLAMMATION

Acute inflammation is a protective response of tissue to irritation, injury, or infection, and is characterized by pain, redness, swelling, and sometimes loss of function. It is, under normal circumstances, beneficial, and helps the body repair the effects of trauma or infection. However, prolonged, excess, or chronic inflammation becomes harmful.

When low-grade invisible inflammation occurs in the very cells that comprise our organ systems, a concept I introduced in my first book, *The Wrinkle Cure* (2000), we are placed at great risk for a host of degenerative, age-related diseases. This is because cells that are attacked by self-generated inflammation will not function properly (meaning that we did something to precipitate a pro-inflammatory response in our cells, thus causing malfunction and sometimes complete breakdown).

In other words, cells respond to the way we treat them. If we keep them healthy and free of injury, if we give them the proper nourishment, they keep us alive and running at top form. If we don't, if we expose them to too much sun, to environmental toxins, to extended periods of stress, or to high-glycemic sugars and starches, the cells will react by producing inflammatory chemicals as a deviation of the normal defense mechanism. And if we mistreat our cells in this way on a regular basis, we can end up with organ system failure and diseases like the ones listed, including metabolic syndrome, which can lead to diabetes and obesity.

This hidden inflammation is a novel and previously unrecognized "missing link" in our obesity epidemic. The goal of the Perricone Weight-Loss Diet is to show you how to decrease this inflammation and prevent future inflammatory responses, thereby eliminating the problem of unwanted weight gain and its serious threat to your overall health, self-esteem, and well-being.

THE ROAD TO DISCOVERY

As a dermatologist, I have had the unique opportunity to actually see the very negative effects of this subclinical inflammation on my patients because, unlike the heart or the liver, the skin is a visible organ. The skin is also an excellent barometer or measurement of our internal health and clearly reflects what is going on inside. This can be something as subtle as a change in ruddiness, or an increased pallor—in fact, physicians can look at the skin and make a diagnosis of internal diseases very accurately.

Many of us think of the skin as simply a cosmetic cover for our body. We pretty much ignore it unless or until something goes wrong, such as a breakout of acne right before a big date.

However, nothing could be further from the truth.

The skin is a very complex and important organ and has many functions, including what is known as **barrier function,** that is, it protects us from the environment. It is the body's first line of defense against germs and harmful toxins. Our skin protects us from the sun and cold, and helps regulate body temperature. But the skin does even more. It is a unique part of the immune system and intimately involved with our central nervous system.

THE BRAIN–BEAUTY CONNECTION

If you have seen my specials on public television or have read my previous books, you have heard me often mention something I call the "the brain–beauty connection." This is a fascinating premise and clearly illustrates the fact that all of our organ systems are in constant "cellular" communication with one another. In other words, the skin talks to the brain, the brain talks to the digestive system, and so on. Who knew? Until very recently, scientists had no idea that the body was one giant telecommunications network! Because this is immensely important in understanding the big picture, I would like to take a minute to review this concept with you.

During medical school, one of the many basic science course requirements was embryology, the branch of biology that deals with the formation, early growth, and development of living organisms. In simpler terms, it is the study of the progress of the fetus from conception to shortly before birth. We learned in embryology that all of the major organs of the body, as well as muscle, bone, and other types of tissue, are all derived from **three basic layers** of tissue within the embryo. I learned that both the skin and the brain were derived from the **same** layer of embryonic tissue. This fascinating discovery encouraged me to look for similarities between the skin and brain, in their structure, structural function, and basic function.

When we studied histology, the branch of anatomy that deals with the minute structure of animal and plant tissues (including the major organ systems) as discernible with the microscope, I could actually (thanks to the microscope) see that the skin did, indeed, have many similarities in structure as the brain. When studying pharmacology, I further observed that when someone was given pharmaceutical agents to treat central nervous system problems, the skin improved along with the brain.

It was also in medical school that I began hypothesizing the inflammation–disease connection. When studying a variety of disease processes under the microscope, I found that there was evidence of inflammation in the arteries in cardiovascular disease, and in the pancreas of people with diabetes.

As my studies progressed to dermatology, I found myself once again studying all disease processes under a microscope. Here I observed the presence of microscopic inflammation around most skin cancers. I also saw evidence of inflammation in aging skin. However, no inflammation was present in skin **that didn't have** the clinical signs of aging. I then observed that skin that had been exposed to the sun displayed a tremendous amount of inflammation when viewed through the lens of my microscope. A clear pattern began to emerge in my mind as I continued my research. I became absolutely convinced that this microinflammation was causing serious and perhaps irreversible damage to our cells. What was particularly alarming was the fact that we cannot feel this microinflammation, nor can we see it with the naked eye. Yet it goes on, day after day, in all of our organ systems, heart, brain, and skin. This damage is cumulative, eventually leading to a host of diseases and chronic degenerative conditions.

Since I was absolutely convinced that inflammation was at the basis of aging and age-related diseases, my next step was to search for a therapeutic intervention. But the big question was, "What is **causing** this low-grade inflammation?" In the skin, it was quite apparent that sunlight triggered an inflammatory cascade; in other words, the sunlight started a chain of events that had a domino effect—one event leading to another until the integrity and very existence of the cell itself was threatened. And of course this turned out to be just one of the causes of inflammation in the skin.

Taking advantage of my dermatological training, I began an intensive study of this inflammatory cascade in the skin produced by sun exposure, as I believed that would serve as a model for chronic inflammation in the other organ systems inflamed by other causes. This proved to be very helpful, as the inflammation in skin cells mimicked the inflammatory pathway in all of our organ systems. Here is a step-by-step depiction of how it works.

1. When we walk out into the sun at high noon on a bright summer day, the sunlight creates a reactive molecule known as a **free radical.** The important point to remember here is the word "reactive"—free radicals cause damage to the cells because they are highly reactive.

2. But free radicals exist for only a nanosecond, leading me to believe that they can do very little direct damage to the cells.

3. Therefore, the free radicals must be acting as a trigger, a catalyst, to set off an inflammatory cascade—i.e., a chain of biochemical events leading to the production of toxic, inflammatory chemicals that attack and degrade cell function in *all* organ systems (for example, when they attack the cardiovascular system, it results in the formation of plaque, leading to the hardening of the arteries and heart attacks).

The good news is that we have some protection from free radicals in the form of enzymes and antioxidants. Most of us are familiar with many antioxidants such as vitamin C, vitamin E, alpha lipoic acid, Coenzyme Q10, and beta-carotene. Our body contains some of these antioxidant systems, whether synthesized by the cell or derived from outer or exogenous sources, such as food.

The bad news is that when we take that walk in the noonday sun, many of the antioxidant systems that are found naturally in our skin, such as vitamin C, Coenzyme Q10, and vitamin E, are depleted very rapidly. And so, within a matter of minutes, the free radicals begin attacking the outside portion of the cell, known as the cell plasma membrane. Antioxidants rush to the scene of the attack, but are quickly used up in the fight. Because our defense mechanisms aren't perfect, the outer, very fragile cell plasma membrane is damaged.

THE MECHANISM OF A VICIOUS CYCLE

What follows the damage to the cell plasma membrane is a kind of domino effect that, in the end, causes a vicious cycle of increased inflammation. Here's how it goes:

◆ The cell plasma membrane is made up of a double layer of fats called a "lipid bi-layer," and this fragile film is easily and rapidly oxidized by the free radicals. This leads to the breakdown of the membrane that produces a substance known as "arachidonic acid."

▼

◆ Arachidonic acid is further oxidized by enzyme systems to produce very active chemical products with pro-inflammatory activity such as "prostaglandins." Arachidonic acid can also leak into the interior of the cell and get into the mitochondria, the tiny furnace used for energy production.

▼

◆ Arachidonic acid then disrupts energy production of the cell, which is critically needed for cellular repair.

▼

◆ The fats in the cell plasma membrane can also become oxidized and mimic chemical messengers in the body, such as platelet-activating factor (PAF), which also triggers a series of inflammatory events on a cellular level.

▼

- All of these events, cumulatively known as "oxidative stress," lead to increased production of free radicals *inside* the cell, with the activation of tiny messengers called transcription factors such as AP-1 and **nuclear factor kappa B,** or **NfkB** for short (we will learn a lot more about these transcription factors throughout this book).

When NfkB detects oxidative stress, it translocates to the nucleus of the cell, which contains the DNA (which in turn contains the master instructions of the cell). NfkB attaches to a portion of the DNA and instructs the cell to make inflammatory chemicals such as interleukins 1 and 6 and Tumor Necrosis Factor, types of cytokines (intercellular chemical messenger proteins released by white blood cells as well as other cells) that create further inflammation and damage.

- When NfkB is activated in skin cells along with another transcription factor called AP-1, it can lead to wrinkles in the skin.

▼

- When NfkB is activated in the brain, it can lead to Alzheimer's disease, and activated in other organs it can lead to cancer.

▼

- When NfkB is activated in the pancreas, it can lead to the destruction of the b cells of the pancreas, which are the sole source of insulin, resulting in diabetes.

▼

- NfkB blocks the ability to utilize insulin effectively, which leads to the storage of body fat, causing us to gain weight and have great difficulty shedding the pounds.

As we can see, once activated, NfkB can wreak havoc. You may be familiar with some of these terms, such as "transcription factor NfkB," because I introduced them first in *The Wrinkle Cure* and later in *The Perricone Prescription*. I am reviewing them here because they are so important in the inflammatory process—and this entire inflammatory progression, from start to finish is, beyond any doubt, a major **precipitating factor** in obesity. This is the phenomenon that will be explained in the next chapter.

Chapter 3

Breaking the Inflammation–Fat Connection

An invasion of armies can be resisted,
but not an idea whose time has come.
— VICTOR HUGO

Now that we have a basic understanding of the dangers of microinflammation, we are going to learn how it contributes to obesity, unwanted weight gain, and difficulty in losing weight. My journey to unlocking the obesity/weight gain dilemma began when I was researching ways to reduce microinflammation in patients seeking to slow down the aging process and decrease their risk of age-related disease.

My early research indicated that food had a tremendous influence on this inflammation and, depending on the foods and beverages we chose, could either increase or decrease inflammation in the body. This led me to develop what I call the "anti-inflammatory diet," the foundation for an internal approach to staying young and living a longer, healthier life. The way to accomplish this is by decreasing the microinflammation that goes on in our cells all day, every day.

As I continued to introduce thousands of patients to the anti-inflammatory diet over the years, I quickly discovered that those patients who had extra body fat rapidly lost weight, as mentioned in the previous chapter. However, there was something else going on as well. None of the people who lost weight looked haggard or tired–symptoms many report when they embark on a weight-loss regimen. On the contrary, these patients following the anti-inflammatory diet looked radiant and felt energized while on the program. Although I was focusing on halting many of the signs of aging, I couldn't help but marvel at this rapid and somewhat unexpected weight loss. As I documented these facts, case by case, I also observed that the patients who faithfully embraced the anti-inflammatory food choices not only experienced a rapid loss of body fat, they were maintaining their muscle tissue.

What was it about this program of eating a wide array of natural, unprocessed, healthy foods that would account for such rapid weight loss in these patients? The anti-inflammatory diet is not an extremely low-calorie diet. In fact, as you shall see later in this book, some of the key components are high-fat fish, such as wild Alaskan salmon. Also recommended are dark green leafy salads dressed with extra virgin olive oil (no diet dressing on my salad!), lots of fresh fruits and vegetables, old-fashioned oatmeal, nuts, seeds, and probiotics such as yogurt and kefir—a veritable cornucopia of delicious, natural foods from all of the major food groups. Not only is it not low calorie, it is not nonfat or low fat. I advocate the liberal use of the "healthy" fats. These include the omega-3 fatty acids found in salmon and the oleic acid found in extra virgin olive oil, which helps us to absorb the omega-3s and other vitamins and nutrients while keeping our cells supple. When you consider that I first developed this program back in the early 1980s, right at the heart of the no-fat mania sweeping America, it seems even more amazing!

But I knew what I knew and I knew what I saw when I looked at inflammation under the microscope. And what I knew was that I needed therapeutic interventions to rapidly reduce inflammation in the body on a cellular level. The anti-inflammatory diet did just that. It was apparent in the healthy glow of the patients on the program, in their energy and brisk step, in their mental clarity and elevated mood, and—could it be—in their rapid shedding of body fat? Could inflammation also be at the very basis of obesity and weight gain? And so my research into this incredible, universal problem began. Not only did I carefully follow many patients with extra weight, whether it was 10 pounds or 200 pounds, I also studied the world's literature for any scrap of information I could find on the link between inflammation and obesity—no matter how seemingly insignificant. I was also totally mystified as to why the anti-inflammatory diet would lead to a rapid loss of body fat *without* losing muscle mass—a detrimental by-product seen in all other weight-reducing diets.

This was of monumental importance because physicians have long been puzzled by the following fact: when people lose a significant amount of body weight, 50 percent of it is muscle mass. This loss of muscle mass is responsible for that drawn, aged appearance of those who have lost weight. The loss of lean muscle mass also decreases overall health in several ways. We must have muscle to perform all of the activities associated with everyday life. Muscle also impacts strength, balance, ability to burn calories, and susceptibility to certain diseases.

And yet, my patients following the anti-inflammatory diet exhibited none of this loss of muscle mass. Why was this? I knew that as a person ages, their body composition changes. I was determined to find the solution to this intriguing puzzle and decided to focus my study on a group of normal, healthy people who lose muscle mass even though they are leading normal, active lives. This group of people is our senior citizens. According to Navinchandra Dadhaniya, M.D., a specialist in geriatric medicine at Illini Hospital, a healthy, young person's body composition includes 30 percent muscle, 20 percent fat, and 10 percent bone. A person age 75 or older may have only 15 percent muscle, 40 percent fat, and 8 percent bone. It is interesting to note that as we age, the muscle loss can be quite profound in some individuals, despite their active lifestyle and apparent physical health.

THE INFLAMMATION–MUSCLE MASS CONNECTION

This loss of muscle mass in older people is called sarcopenia. I wondered if I could use sarcopenia as a model to measure and compare the muscle mass loss seen in those who diet. I was fascinated to find that patients who suffered from sarcopenia had **higher** circulating levels of inflammatory markers than those who experienced less muscle mass loss, while other parameters had insignificant differences. These other parameters, such as levels of growth hormones and sex hormones, were fairly close to the same level in both groups. In other words, those subjects with the greatest loss of muscle mass were in an **inflammatory** state. These inflammatory markers, such as C-reactive protein and cytokines such as interleukin-6, are elevated in those people who suffer the most muscle mass loss or severe sarcopenia.

So here it was again, rearing its ugly head: low-grade, invisible inflammation as a causative factor in age-related muscle loss. I was now very much intrigued by the possibility that age-related muscle mass loss could be used as a model for the muscle loss seen in patients who were losing muscle with their weight reduction diets. But I had seen firsthand that by following my anti-inflammatory diet, patients were able to lose significant amounts of weight *without* the corresponding loss of muscle.

Could the answer be that inflammation is at the basis of muscle loss during the dieting process?

I thought the connection was an interesting supposition, but first I had to complete my research into inflammation and obesity. Scientists have discovered an alarming property of fat cells—one that was not known until very recently. They discovered that fat cells are rather unique in that they are not inert, but highly active little devils.

THE TRUTH ABOUT BODY FAT

This past decade has seen a complete turnaround in the way scientists regard white adipose tissue—better known as **body fat.** They no longer look upon it as an inert deposit of fat cells, stored as the result of overeating. They now realize that areas of fat storage are actually an **active endocrine organ. Fat produces hormones** as do our pancreas, thyroid, parathyroid, adrenals, pineal, pituitary, and testes/ovaries, the organs that comprise the endocrine system. We are beginning to define body fat as a group of cells communicating with other organ systems such as the brain, the liver, the bone marrow, skeletal muscle, the adrenal cortex, the sympathetic nervous system, and the complete immune system. And the message they are communicating is not good.

This is extremely important because the **body fat itself** controls how much body fat is going to be stored. It also affects our appetite, our energy expenditure, and our immune system. Body fat accomplishes this by secreting hormones known as **adipokines.** Adipokines are proteins that act as messengers throughout the body (more examples of the communications network). Like certain types of cytokines, those chemical messengers that have pro-inflammatory activity, adipokines can contribute to systemic, low-grade, chronic inflammation.

This becomes even more frightening when we begin to understand that the greater amount of fat we have stored, the greater its negative influence on the entire body, an extremely destructive, inflammatory influence.

In fact, it would not be too great a stretch to compare excess body fat storage to a tumor, for several valid reasons. A large store of body fat can be so overwhelming to the system that the fat cells have to secrete hormone-like substances to increase blood vessel growth necessary to feed the accumulation of fat. In addition, like a tumor, blood vessel growth cannot keep up with the rapidly growing mass of fat cells, which then begin to become oxygen-starved. These oxygen-starved cells start releasing inflammatory chemicals to further trigger blood vessel growth. These same events are seen in tumor growth, as well.

I realize that this tumor comparison may sound radical and somewhat alarming. However, we need to realize that I am making this comparison to illustrate that excess body fat is not a cosmetic, benign occurrence, giving the false impression of a fat but otherwise healthy and happy person. This active group of cells is creating a spectrum of problems in every organ system, from bone growth to sexual reproduction. This agglomeration of fat cells, now an active endocrine organ, has the unique distinction of being the **only** endocrine organ to send pro-inflammatory and destructive signals to all organ systems throughout the body.

WHY DO WE LOSE MUSCLE?

When we are obese there is a constant exchange of fat for muscle. However, this is greatly accelerated when we are dieting. One reason is that we tend to have a markedly reduced caloric intake compared to when we are not dieting. Most overweight people, especially the obese, have chronic high levels of insulin that will begin to drop as soon as they start dieting. This is a two-edged sword, as low insulin levels decrease inflammation, which allows us to utilize body fat for energy. However, insulin is required to bring protein into the cells to maintain muscle mass. The overweight or obese person has cells that are insensitive to insulin due to their chronic high levels. That is, their body is so used to the overly high levels, it cannot recognize these new lower levels, thus it is unable to trigger the amino acid uptake needed to maintain muscle mass (insulin is needed to take up both sugar and amino acids into the muscle).

This is why it is critical to take a powerful anti-inflammatory approach to dieting. Remember, it is the inflammatory chemicals, such as NfkB, that block the effects of insulin—whether it is to metabolize blood sugar or to nourish muscles with amino acids. Overexercising can further put us into a catabolic state (in which complex molecules are broken down into simpler ones) because of the higher requirement of nutrients needed for active muscles.

We have long known that having extra weight also increases our risk of type 2 diabetes. Researchers have been searching for the common factor between low-grade inflammation, weight gain, and type 2 diabetes. They know that people with extra

Inflammation, Body Fat, and Heart Disease

Scientists and physicians now recognize that heart disease is mediated by inflammatory chemicals. In fact, forward thinking cardiologists are now measuring C-reactive protein, a marker of inflammation, to identify patients at risk for heart disease. This is proving to be significantly more accurate than looking at cholesterol. In fact, many cardiologists now report that elevated C-reactive protein is four times more accurate in predicting heart disease than elevated cholesterol.

C-reactive protein is a special type of protein produced in high amounts by the liver during episodes of acute inflammation. High circulating levels of C-reactive protein also indicate stomach inflammation. Researchers at UC Davis recently found that endothelial cells (the delicate lining of the circulatory system) also produce C-reactive protein, a key finding that helps to explain how plaque formation is initiated. This is particularly important because endothelial cells are supposed to **protect** the arteries from the effects of C-reactive protein. Researchers also found that C-reactive protein can cause these endothelial cells in our arteries to produce a substance called plasminogen activator inhibitor, which leads to blood clot formation. C-reactive protein can also lead to activation of white blood cells in the lining of the arteries to promote plaque formation. These findings begin to explain why those individuals with excess body fat are at a higher risk for cardiovascular disease. Scientists have discovered that excess weight leads to low-grade chronic inflammation; low-grade, chronic inflammation leads to mildly elevated C-reactive protein, which can lead to heart disease.

body fat have higher levels of inflammatory markers such as C-reactive protein and some of the interleukins. Now they began to turn their attention to the role of transcription factors in obesity. They found that the transcription factor NfkB is activated in obese individuals, as discussed in the previous chapter.

However, it gets even worse. Elevated NfkB is also directly responsible for a condition known as "insulin resistance." When we are insulin resistant, our insulin mechanism does not work well—we do not use insulin properly. This results in elevated levels of both insulin and blood sugar, raising the risk of developing type 2 diabetes.

Don't Get "Waisted"

How do we know if we are insulin resistant or may become so in the future? Scientists have found that without a doubt, our waist size is a good indicator of a person's risk of insulin resistance—an early stage in the development of diabetes and heart disease. The size of our waist has already been recognized as an indicator of the possible development of cardiovascular disease, but scientists in Sweden have found that it can also be used to measure our sensitivity to insulin.

"A waist circumference of less than 39 inches reduces the risk of individuals of both sexes from being at risk of insulin resistance," Hans Wahrenberg, of the Karolinska University Hospital in Stockholm, said in a study reported online by the *British Medical Journal.*

If you are starting to store weight around the middle, be aware that the ramifications are much more than aesthetic or the letting out of your belt a notch or two or three. You are increasing your risk of both diabetes and heart attack. Fortunately, the Perricone Weight-Loss Diet has strategies to combat this.

PUTTING IT ALL TOGETHER

What happens (besides elevating our risk for disease) when people who are carrying excess fat have elevated levels of NfkB?

- It interferes with the body's ability to use insulin
- increasing our blood sugar levels,
- which then further increases inflammation
- and makes us store body fat.

High levels of insulin circulating in our bloodstream keeps us fat because it inhibits the production of an enzyme that breaks down body fat for fuel. In addition, we cannot access this body fat for energy. It also causes us to be hungry all of the time.

To recap, remember this simple formula. When we eat sugars and foods that are rapidly converted to sugar, they cause a rapid rise in blood sugar, resulting in the release of high levels of insulin into the bloodstream. This causes weight gain via two factors.

1. Your body's principal way of getting rid of sugar (which is toxic) is to burn it. The sugar that your body can't burn will be stored as glycogen.
2. When your glycogen reserves are full, the excess sugar gets stored as fat. If you continue to eat sugar, your body will burn it up, stopping you from burning up fat—and so it goes.

We have now learned that

- transcription factor NfkB is a strong marker for and possible cause of insulin resistance
- c-reactive protein is also elevated in people with insulin resistance

Now I was beginning to pull together all the pieces of the puzzle:

- Inflammation is measurably elevated in people with excess weight.
- Inflammation is responsible for our inability to utilize insulin and blood sugar for energy.
- The inability to utilize insulin and blood sugar effectively leads to the storage of fat.
- Stored fat cells act as a veritable factory for creating inflammatory chemicals.
- These chemicals increase inflammation.
- Increased inflammation inhibits insulin and energy usage and causes the accumulation of additional excess fat.

HOW DO WE BREAK THE CYCLE?

As the pieces of the puzzle began to come together, I began to understand why people were losing weight on my anti-inflammatory diet. The foods and supplements that I had been recommending to reduce wrinkles and slow down the aging process were also inhibiting the inflammation that causes insulin resistance and body fat storage. As mentioned, I advocated eating ample quantities of cold-water fish like wild Alaskan salmon, sardines, anchovies, mackerel, herring, shad, and trout—ideally one fish meal per day. I also strongly recommended the use of nutritional supplements like omega-3 fish oil, alpha lipoic acid, carnitine, CLA (conjugated linoleic acid), glutamine, Coenzyme Q10, astaxanthin, and dimethylaminoethanol (DMAE) (more about these in Chapter 6).

Why are these foods and supplements so effective? Because they all have high anti-inflammatory properties. Brightly colored fruits and vegetables signal the presence of antioxidants, Nature's natural anti-inflammatories. Wild Alaskan salmon also contains a powerful antioxidant, anti-inflammatory (responsible for its deep pink/red coloring) known as astaxanthin, reported to be more than one hundred times stronger than vitamins C and E combined. Further, I realized that the single most powerful causative agent for reducing inflammation was the high levels of essential fats that I was recommending. These fats, particularly the omega-3 essential fatty acids found in high-fat fish and fish oil, act as powerful, natural anti-inflammatories.

Recognizing that a great many Americans were overweight, and their diets were practically devoid of the omega-3s, I asked myself the following questions:

Could it be that *low* levels of the essential fatty acids *exacerbate inflammation* and promote weight gain? And could it then be that *high* levels of essential fatty acids also *reduce the inflammation* that is found in people with excess body fat, thereby accelerating that loss?

Perhaps we can find the answer in the huge increase of overweight people that has its roots in the no-fat and low-fat craze of the 1980s and continues to escalate to this day. Women in particular have suffered from the ridiculous and dangerous notion that all fat is bad and must be avoided at all costs. Not only did they **not** lose weight, this dangerous fad accelerated the development of wrinkles and contributed to an epidemic of mental depression and obesity.

The reason for this is twofold. First, the onset of the low-fat diet deprived brain cells of the critically essential healthy fat needed for normal brain function. When I say "normal" brain function, I refer to the production of those important chemical messengers known as "neurotransmitters" that allow brain cells to communicate with one another. We all know from television and magazines that low levels of serotonin, the classic "feel good" neurotransmitter, can lead to chronic depression. By depriving the brain of the healthy fats it needs to produce serotonin and other neurotransmitters, we are effectively opening the door to depression and a host of other mental, behavioral, neurological, and psychological maladies.

Second, in addition to the damage done by the deprivation of healthy fats, the 1980s saw the rise in the ingestion of massive quantities of fat-free, high-glycemic car-

Adult-onset Diabetes Breaks the Age Barrier

Perhaps the most alarming aspect of the current state of diabetes is the incidence of type 2 diabetes appearing in young children and teens. This increase is so startling that it is being called an epidemic. Type 2 diabetes, which used to be called adult-onset diabetes, occurs when the body doesn't produce enough insulin or loses its ability to efficiently use insulin. Until recently, it was usually diagnosed only in adults over the age of 30.

Amazingly, many researchers profess to be mystified as to this phenomenon and do not yet fully understand the reasons for such a change. However, if you look at the increase in fast-food consumption (consisting mainly of high-glycemic French fries and burger buns, burgers high in pro-inflammatory saturated fats, super-size sodas), the influx of high fructose corn syrup into a huge array of food and beverages, the rise of a sedentary lifestyle thanks to the video game and PC—the proliferation of high-glycemic carbohydrates—it becomes clear where the responsibility for this epidemic lies: a 24/7 inflammatory lifestyle.

bohydrates, such as the ubiquitous rice or corn cake, baked potato chips, nonfat cookies, and so on, which has played a significant role in the epidemic of both obesity and type 2 diabetes.

When we eat these high-glycemic carbohydrates, we deplete our precious reserves of serotonin. For example, a breakfast consisting of a low-fat muffin or bagel with fat-free cream cheese and jam, and a glass of fruit juice, will cause a rapid rise in blood sugar. This results in a release of serotonin in the brain, giving us a warm, fuzzy feeling as the carbohydrates are rapidly converted to glucose (sugar) by our digestive system. High levels of sugar are now circulating in our bloodstream, which signals the pancreas to secrete insulin to help bring down these high levels of sugar. The problem begins when the insulin pushes the blood sugar levels down to levels too low. The result is a rapid decline in serotonin levels, a quick drop in energy—and an almost irresistible craving for more sugar and carbs.

In other words, we need another "fix" in order to get back the warm, fuzzy feeling. In fact, many women "self-medicate" with high-glycemic carbs in their rational desire to simply feel good. I say "women" here because women generally tend to have lower levels of serotonin than men. And these levels drop even lower during parts of the menstrual cycle and when they are postmenopausal. To compensate for this, women resort to consuming larger amounts of high-glycemic carbohydrates than their male counterparts. Since many women place themselves on calorie-restricted diets, they then tend to forgo healthy proteins and healthy fats to make up for the calories contained in the carbohydrates.

This often results in women looking older than men of their same age group, because healthy fats and protein are necessary for cellular repair, while high-carb diets accelerate the aging process. The fluctuating blood sugar and insulin levels place them in a constant battle with excess weight gain, while the depletion of their serotonin leaves women at greater risk for depression (it is no coincidence that Prozac, a prescription antidepressant that elevates serotonin levels, first came to attention during this decade of high carb/low-fat diets).

This sorry state of affairs is contributing to the breakdown of the mental and physical health of men, women, and children at an escalating rate. We are overweight, we are depressed, we are fatigued, and we are stressed. And more and more of us, children and adults alike, are turning to chemical and pharmacological solutions to the problem. However, these "solutions" treat the symptom while ignoring the underlying problem. There is a better way.

AN "ELEGANT" SOLUTION

In science and mathematics, we use the term **elegant** to describe an experiment, invention, discovery, or concept that combines simplicity, power, and a certain ineffable grace of design. To me, there is no discovery more elegant, simple, or powerful than the discovery of fish oil and its restorative properties. The omega-3 essential fatty acids found in the high-fat fish and in fish oil can accelerate the loss of fat and elevate serotonin levels as well. This method is far superior than trying to alter brain chemicals with prescription antidepressants. The only "side effects" of omega-3s when taken at the recommended doses are

- loss of body fat
- maintenance of muscle mass
- elevated mood
- improved attention span
- stabilized blood sugar levels

- lowered insulin levels
- healthy serotonin levels
- loss of the roller-coaster effects of the carbohydrate highs and lows
- decreased appetite
- increased radiance to skin
- healthier immune system
- increased energy levels
- decreased symptoms and severity of rheumatoid arthritis
- reduced symptoms and severity of chronic skin conditions such as eczema
- decreased cardiovascular risk

In the next chapter, you will learn more about the miracle of the omega-3s. And while we cannot place all of our physical and mental ills on the lack of this important nutrient, we can certainly come close. These essential fats, long missing from our refined, overprocessed diets just may prove to be the fundamental missing link in winning our fight against obesity.

Chapter 4

The Omega-3 Weight-Loss Miracle

A scientific truth does not triumph by convincing its opponents and making them see the light, but rather because its opponents eventually die and a new generation grows up that is familiar with it.

— MAX PLANCK

The concepts you have learned in the last two chapters are important to understand so that you can make informed decisions about your diet and health. However, if there is one concept you take away from this book, it should be the importance of a diet rich in anti-inflammatory essential fatty acids—especially the one known as omega-3.

Here's why: We all know that in order to lose weight we have to reduce the number of calories we take in and/or increase the number of calories we burn off. When we take in more calories than we need, the excess gets stored as body fat. Omega-3 fatty acids help us burn off those calories before they get a chance to "sit around in storage"—which means we will end up carrying less excess weight.

Here's what you need to do: **increase** your intake of omega-3 (through foods and supplements I'll tell you about later) and **decrease** your intake of pro-inflammatory high-glycemic carbohydrates (sugars and starches) and saturated fats (found in most fried foods, full-fat dairy products, and meat).

This simple increase/decrease formula will not only improve your overall health—nourishing the skin, hair, mucous membranes, nerves, and glands, and help to prevent cardiovascular disease—it will inhibit the conversion of calories into body fat. In addition, these essential fats encourage the body to burn calories as body heat and increase its sensitivity to insulin, thereby preventing storage of body fat and reducing the risk of diabetes and obesity.

One of the goals of the Perricone Weight-Loss Diet is to restore the proper ratio of essential fatty acids, particularly omega-3.

TURNING UP THE HEAT

While I was a college student I really wanted to gain weight and put on muscle—to overcome the 98-pound weakling appearance. In order to achieve this, I read a lot of literature written by body-building experts. In addition to beginning a rigorous weight training program, I arbitrarily decided to increase my daily caloric intake to 7,000 calories. I very quickly began to increase my strength and muscle mass, but surprisingly not my body fat.

One of the distinct things I noticed was that my body would produce a lot of heat after eating a meal. In fact I threw off so much body heat, my girlfriend remarked that it was uncomfortable to sit next to me. I was very intrigued by this process and I started searching for the cause. I quickly discovered that this is what physicians refer to as "postprandial thermogenesis"—which simply means "the generation or production of heat following a meal," although in my case it was somewhat exaggerated.

As the years went by, I continued my exercise routine and ate essentially half the calories with some important improvements. However, I found that I produced far less heat after a meal than I had when I was younger. I also noticed that it was becoming increasingly difficult to stay lean. I learned that this was not unusual. The younger we are, the greater the postprandial thermogenesis. I was quite curious as to the mechanism of this process.

I soon learned that when you consume food, its energy (measured as calories) can take one of two paths in the body:

♦ Food calories can be burned in the mitochondria for production of ATP (adenosine triphosphate), a high-energy phosphate molecule used to store and release energy for work within the body. This entire process is known as "oxidative phosphorylation."

▼

♦ More often as we get older, the food can go on to be stored as body fat (triglycerides in adipose tissue) or stored as glycogen in the liver and muscles (glycogen is the form in which foods are stored in the body as energy). If we can "uncouple" the oxidation from the phosphorylation, food calories can be burned off by thermogenesis. Thermogenesis bypasses the ATP-mediated energy. If the majority of food we ate was transformed into body heat we would stay slim and trim.

It is probably no coincidence that overweight people have very little postprandial thermogenesis.

This inspired me to search for an agent that would "uncouple" the making of ATP (oxidative phosphorylation) from food so that the food we ate was burned up as heat.

I eagerly began a quest to discover the ultimate uncoupling agent. I was soon to learn that, unfortunately, the best uncouplers had undesirable side effects or were highly toxic. In fact, one of the most efficient uncoupling agents is ephedrine (extracted from the ancient Chinese medicinal herb ephedra), which was a popular ingredient in various diet formulations. However, ephedrine, which was banned by the FDA in 2004, has stimulant effects on the central nervous system and heart and has been linked to high blood pressure, heart palpitations, and other damaging side effects.

I soon gave up my quest for the ultimate uncoupling drug or dietary supplement. I began to focus my research on strategies to reduce inflammation in the body, which I firmly believed to be a causative factor in many diseases. I discovered that food has a tremendous influence on this inflammation—it can either increase or decrease inflammation in the body.

This research led me to create the anti-inflammatory diet, where I discovered that the omega-3 essential fatty acids (EFAs) were powerful anti-inflammatories. Little did I know that my discoveries would far surpass my wildest, earlier quests.

One important role of EFAs turned out to be their effect on insulin levels. High levels of insulin are pro-inflammatory; this is one of the reasons people gain excess weight and cannot seem to lose it when they diet. Chronically high levels create an "insensitivity" to the insulin. Excess insulin continues to be released into the bloodstream, resulting in the storage of fat.

When we add omega-3 essential fatty acids to our diets, we begin to "sensitize" our cells to insulin. Insulin receptors are found in the cell's plasma membrane, which controls the passage of substances in and out of the cell. Essential fatty acids keep this critical and fragile portion of the cell flexible, thereby keeping these receptors intact and sensitive to fluctuations in insulin levels. The correct balance of dietary EFAs enables the receptors to respond to even small amounts of insulin, helping us to maintain healthy blood sugar levels and ensure an adequate uptake of sugar and amino acids into cells to build muscle and minimize fat storage.

I then discovered that the essential fatty acids found in cold-water, high-fat fish and fish oil possess a number of even more astonishing properties. These essential fats, particularly the omega-3s, are extremely important in energy production within the mitochondria. Omega-3 EFAs also inhibit the production of the enzyme fatty acid synthase, which plays a role in the storage of calories as body fat. In addition, the essential fatty acids are responsible for a phenomenon known as "fuel partitioning."

When fuel partitioning is working efficiently, EFAs direct our bodies to store carbohydrates in the form of glycogen, rather than as hard-to-lose body fat. Glycogen is mainly stored in the liver and muscles and releases sugar (glucose) into the blood when needed by cells. It is the chief source of stored fuel in the body, and is the first place the body turns to when it needs quick energy between meals or when energy needs cannot be met by food intake alone, such as during intensive bouts of physical or mental activity. It is the glycogen stored in the muscle that directly affects how hard and how long we can exercise. In short, omega-3s facilitate the temporary storage of calories as glycogen, which is used for immediate energy needs, while encouraging the burning of stored body fat.

The most exciting moment of my quest, however, has to be when I came across a groundbreaking study that held the long-awaited answer I had been searching for—clear evidence that omega-3 fatty acids can **increase thermogenesis,** thereby dissipating calories in the form of increased body heat, instead of storing them as body fat. Ongoing research suggests that EFAs may be able to directly influence important metabolic genes in our cells—genes that control how we synthesize glycogen and how we store and burn fat. This may be due to a steroidlike substance in our bodies called PPARs (perixosome proliferator-activated receptors), which, when bound to fats like EFAs, can "switch on" key genes involved in burning fat. Further research also suggests that omega-3s switch on a protein called uncoupling protein-3, which plays an important part in energy metabolism. Higher levels of uncoupling proteins result in more energy being dissipated as heat, increasing energy expenditure and decreasing stored fat. This is a critical function because stored body fat is very difficult to lose, as millions of unsuccessful dieters know. Could omega-3s be the uncoupling agent I had been searching for?

NUTRITIONAL FACTORS HOLD THE KEY

Amazingly, it seems that we don't need some new superdrug as the solution to the weight loss problem. **For the first time, science had proven beyond a doubt that nutritional components of our diet can directly control and influence key metabolic genes in our cells.** That means the EFAs we consume can significantly affect the way we store and burn fat. This nutritional aspect was particularly compelling because it meant that the effects would be physiological—that is, they would work with the body, as opposed to against it, the way a drug would. This also meant that the positive, beneficial effects of these essential fatty acids would always have efficacy; unlike a drug, we would not build up a tolerance or resistance to their therapeutic properties. These omega-3 fatty acids would always be on the job, helping us to burn excess fat, while simultaneously decreasing our propensity for fat storage.

Omega-3 is not the only type of essential fatty acid pertinent to our discussion. There is also omega-6. Both types are needed to form and maintain the structural and functional integrity of cell membranes, provide fuel for cellular energy, and create the hormone-like messenger chemicals, the prostaglandins and the eicosanoids, which regulate many key metabolic functions.

Because the body cannot make these essential fats, we must obtain them from our diets. This is a lot easier said than done. For one thing, many of us consume a low ratio of essential fatty acids compared to our intake of saturated fatty acids, such as those found in full-fat dairy products and meat (we all know that saturated fats are pro-inflammatory and are associated with an increased risk of cardiovascular disease).

Unfortunately, when most of us do consume essential fatty acids, they tend to be omega-6, which is found in grains and vegetable oils such as corn and safflower. In fact, very few of us are getting the proper ratio of omega-3 to omega-6, which may account for the growing prevalence of serious health conditions like heart attacks, cancer, asthma, lupus, schizophrenia, depression, accelerated aging, ADHD (attention deficit/hyperactivity disorder), Alzheimer's disease, metabolic syndrome, obesity, and diabetes in our society.

Skye's Story

It was a blustery late spring day when I got the call from Brad (not his real name), a well-known fitness trainer to many of Hollywood's most famous actors and actresses. "I've got a challenge on my hands and a deadline looming," Brad explained. "I'm working with Skye (not her real name) on a new action film. My challenge is to get her into the 'action hero' shape that the role requires. Her last film required her to gain a lot of extra weight and now we've got to get it off in record time."

Her last role was as a 30-something desperate housewife whose husband's passionate affairs outside of the marriage plunged her into a depression. Her character retaliated by starting an equally passionate affair, although hers was with Häagen-Dazs and Mallomars. By the end of the film she had gained a solid twenty pounds on her abdomen, hips, and thighs.

"Skye has been following a low-calorie, low-fat diet," Brad told me, "and we have a pretty grueling workout schedule. She's lost ten pounds and her musculature is good, but we've still got a way to go, and not a lot of time to get there. Shooting starts in two weeks." To make matters worse, Brad confided, "Skye is feeling depressed and frustrated."

I carefully went over Skye's daily meal plan and exercise routine and a clear picture began to emerge. She was drinking a lot of coffee and her diet contained no detectable levels of omega-3 essential fatty acids. Without these omega-3s it was just about impossible for Skye to properly metabolize fat. I set up an anti-inflammatory routine for Skye to follow, so

that she could lose the weight and maintain the all-important muscle. After all, what is an action hero without muscle!

I started her on three 1,000 mg omega-3 fish oil capsules to be taken three times per day—a whopping total of 9,000 mg per day. This may seem extreme, but the circumstances called for it. *In addition, I suggested she take 1,000 mg of acetyl-L-carnitine and 2,000 mg of CLA per day.*

I also sent Skye a case of canned wild Alaskan sockeye salmon and advised her to eat a can a day for lunch along with a dark green salad and an apple. I advised her to purchase eggs from free-range chickens whose diet was high in flax; these eggs were another good source of omega-3s. For dinner I recommended that she eat cold-water fish, such as salmon, at least five nights per week—again with a dark green leafy salad dressed with lemon juice and extra virgin olive oil, with either an apple or grapefruit for dessert. Admittedly this was a pretty strict regimen, but we needed to accomplish a small miracle in a short amount of time.

I told her to drink six to eight 8-ounce glasses of water per day, and to eliminate the coffee and substitute green tea. The green tea would not only help her burn fat, it would give her a feeling of well-being. The salmon and fish oil would also go a long way toward lifting her depression. At the end of the first week, Brad phoned with an update on Skye's progress. She had dropped five pounds, her mood was excellent, her motivation was back, and amazingly, she was making

This imbalance upsets the proverbial fat-metabolizing apple cart. An overabundance of omega-6 is inflammatory and interferes with the body's ability to use omega-3s—a serious situation because of the positive effects of omega-3s we talked about earlier: they inhibit the calories we consume from being stored as body fat, while promoting the burning of body fat we already have.

OMEGA-3: THE INSIDE STORY

The body needs two components of omega-3s, DHA (docosahexaenoic acid) and EPA (eicosapentaenoic acid). The healthiest food sources of DHA and EPA are fish— especially fatty cold-water species such as salmon (and other fish you'll learn about in the next chapter), shellfish, seaweed, and algae. But what happens if these sea-based foods are not available? We can survive without seafood because the body can make EPA and DHA from alpha linolenic acid (ALA), the omega-3 fatty acid found primarily in unrefined whole grains, dark, leafy greens, and certain nuts and seeds (mainly flaxseed, pumpkin seeds, walnuts, hemp seeds, and the oils extracted from them— especially flax).

How Omega-3s Aid Weight Control

As you can see, essential fatty acids affect and trigger a number of different obesity-fighting processes. Here is a short but comprehensive overview of what they are and what they do:

- *Reduce inflammation* that promotes weight gain.
- *Enable burning of dietary fats* by transporting fatty acids into the mitochondria of our cells for burning as fuel.
- *Enhance "fuel efficiency"* by exerting positive influences on the process of fuel partitioning.
- *Improve blood sugar control* by sensitizing our cells and enabling receptors to respond to even small amounts of insulin.[1]
- *Stimulate the secretion of leptin,* a peptide hormone that is produced by fat cells. Leptin acts on the hypothalamus to suppress appetite and burn fat stored in adipose tissue (fat cells).
- *Improve fatty acid balance* by reducing conversion of dietary omega-6 EFAs to arachidonic acid (as described in Chapter 2).

- *Influence key anti-obesity genetic switches* (nuclear transcription factors) that govern both inflammation and conversion of food to body fat. They

1. Activate perixosome proliferator-activated receptors (PPARs), which increases the burning of body fat, increases thermogenesis, increases insulin sensitivity, and decreases levels of inflammation.
2. Prevent activation of NfkB.
3. Omega-3 (and omega-6) block the release of sterol response element binding protein-1 (SREBP-1), which switches on the gene that codes for fatty-acid synthase, an enzyme that helps create body fat.

- Omega-3 and omega-6 enhance the body's ability to transport glucose from our blood to our cells via an "insulin-responsive transporter" called GLUT4; they do this by optimizing the fluidity of cell membranes.

---

[1] While omega-3s enhance blood sugar control over the long term, they can raise insulin levels and thereby destabilize blood sugar control temporarily, as the body adjusts. Accordingly, to avoid problems, diabetics should take supplemental omega-3s under the supervision of a physician and monitor blood sugar closely until it restabilizes.

However, the aforementioned seafood starts to look like the ideal choice when we recognize that the body converts only about 15 percent of dietary ALA to EPA, and converts much less to DHA, even under optimal conditions. Worse, the process of converting ALA to EPA and DHA is hampered by factors common to many Americans; an excess of dietary omega-6 fatty acids, an excess of dietary trans-fatty acids (found in many processed and fast foods), diabetes, and excessive alcohol intake. And so, while it is possible to access omega-3s through plant foods, it is less than optimal. When we eat the cold-water fish and take fish oil supplementation we are assured that we are getting the critical omega-3s in a way that allows our bodies to utilize them for the highest benefit.

ANOTHER AMAZING DISCOVERY ABOUT OMEGA-3

There is one other amazing aspect of omega-3s I really wanted to include in this chapter, and it has to do with the use of steroids. This is a subject that is constantly in the news, from professional athletes who break the rules of the game to enhance their performance, to high school boys who give in to peer pressure in order to bulk up and improve their athletic abilities, to young girls and women taking steroids in their quest to be thin and to achieve the "sculpted" look.

Steroids can be terribly dangerous. The major side effects from abusing anabolic steroids can include liver tumors and cancer, jaundice (yellowish pigmentation of skin, tissues, and body fluids), fluid retention, high blood pressure, increases in LDL (bad cholesterol), and decreases in HDL (good cholesterol). Other side effects include kidney tumors, severe acne, trembling, mood swings, and "roid rage."

What steroid users don't know is that omega-3 essential fatty acids can deliver the effects they want–significantly improve athletic performance, helping to make muscle cells stronger and more efficient; actually build muscle and lose body fat–without the dangerous side effects. There are even steroidlike substances in the body, like PPARs mentioned earlier, that can help achieve these goals when activated by omega-3. Matt's story (see p. 38) is a perfect illustration of this healthy alternative.

I have long believed that a holistic, natural solution to any problem should always be our first course of action. Matt's tremendous success once again proved how powerful anti-inflammatory foods and supplements (with omega-3 perhaps topping the

Matt's Story

When I first met Matt he was in serious need of immediate help. Matt's father worked for a major international oil company. Matt had grown up overseas, first
in the Middle East and more recently in Venezuela. It
was a sheltered existence, in which his only friends
were the sons and daughters of the oil company's em-
ployees. His father was called back to the United
States the summer before Matt was to enter his junior
year in high school. His parents enrolled him in a prep
school where excelling in sports, especially football,
was the single most important criteria for popularity.

That summer Matt embarked on a vigorous program of weight lifting with the hope of bulking up his
frame. As the school year started, Matt was delighted
to learn that he had made the team. But there was a
dark side to this victory. Matt had developed a pretty
severe case of acne. In addition, the captain of the
football team had recently returned from a summer
vacation in Mexico, where anabolic steroids were both
cheap and plentiful. He came back well-supplied and
promptly distributed these drugs to the team.

The acne breakouts had driven Matt to my office
door, and as he detailed his recent history, I felt confident that I could help him. After practice, Matt and
his teammates would descend on the nearest fast-
food emporium, where they would slake their thirst
with 32-ounce sodas and enjoy triple cheeseburgers
with large orders of fries. He confessed that he was
starting to develop excess fat around his waistline.

Matt also confided his anxiety about the steroids—
he had heard that they were not only dangerous, but

could also make his acne worse. I explained to Matt
that lifting weights can increase the circulating levels
of the male hormone testosterone because that is the
body's natural way of increasing muscle mass and re-
pairing muscle. This testosterone can also make acne
worse—but fortunately there are ways to control it.
Conversely, taking an unnatural drug, such as anabolic steroids, has many short- and long-term dangerous side effects—not the least of which is a
worsening of the acne.

"Matt, if you give me a chance, I can not only eliminate your acne," I said, "I can significantly improve
your athletic performance, increase your muscle
mass, and eliminate that excess body fat—without
anabolic steroids.

"First we have to start with the foods you eat.
You're going to have to eliminate all the fast foods,
sodas, and chips from your diet." Matt was not over-
joyed, but he was smart enough to realize that he
needed to take some responsibility for both his acne
and unwanted layer of body fat. For starters, I recommended that the copious amounts of soda needed to
be replaced with pure spring water. Then, I put Matt on
the anti-inflammatory diet. Luckily, Matt loved fish,
which gave me great hopes for a successful outcome. I
recommended that he buy wild Alaskan salmon in cans
for convenience and ideally eat salmon at least five
times per week. In addition to eating liberal amounts
of fresh vegetables and fruits, he needed to start taking high-quality fish oil capsules—1,000 mg per capsule, three per meal, three times a day, for a total of

nine per day (I don't recommend this amount for every-one; always check with a health professional before taking any supplements yourself).

In addition to the fish oil capsules, I also put Matt on the following supplemental regimen, to help increase cellular energy level, provide antioxidant/anti-inflammatory protection, and help facilitate fat loss:

- Carnitine
- Acetyl-L-carnitine
- Alpha lipoic acid
- DMAE
- Conjugated Linoleic Acid (CLA)
- Glutamine
- Chromium Polynicotinate
- Gamma Linoleic Acid (GLA)
- Coenzyme Q10
- Astaxanthin

About three weeks later, I was sitting out on the deck enjoying the view of a tranquil, early October Long Island Sound. As I opened the local Sunday newspaper, I was shocked to read that a group of athletes had been busted for steroid use. As I read on, I recognized that it had happened at Matt's prep school. Since the students were underage their names were not printed, and I inwardly prayed that Matt was not one of the guilty ones.

On Monday my assistant walked into my office and told me that Matt was on the phone and it was urgent. As I answered, I heard Matt's voice, breathless with anxiety. "Doc, it's me, Matt. I want to thank you personally for saving me from this disaster." He told me that he had stopped taking steroids and had faithfully followed the regimen I had set up for him, and the results had been staggering. Within a week, the layer of body fat was gone. His acne lesions were slowly fading and new ones were not forming. Perhaps most exciting was his sense of physical well-being and strength. Matt was rapidly earning the reputation as the most valuable player of the entire team—both for his athletic prowess and his stamina.

list) are to our physical and mental well-being. Best of all, this program works for everyone, regardless of age or gender.

When you eat inflammatory foods your body enters a state of constant, cellular inflammation. Weight loss will be difficult; the processes of aging will accelerate greatly. The key to solving the weight loss enigma is clear: stop cellular inflammation at its dietary source and excess body fat will be eliminated almost automatically (provided caloric intake is in balance with energy expenditure: no approach can work if you consume substantially more calories than you burn during daily activities).

It's important to realize that the processes described here do not happen overnight. As soon as you begin taking in omega-3s (from foods and/or supplements), they start exerting their anti-inflammatory effects. It does take time, however, for EFAs to influence your thermogenesis and fuel partitioning, which is why I recommend that you do not delay introducing omega-3s into your diet. The reason that traditional low-calorie diets fail is that they lack omega-3s, which are essential for healthy metabolism. If you follow the anti-inflammatory diet and ensure the intake of plenty of omega-3 fatty acids, you will successfully lose weight. The powerful anti-inflammatory properties of the omega-3 essential fatty acids hold the key to the weight-control puzzle.

The Perricone Weight-Loss Diet has been carefully developed to accomplish the following goals:

- reduce inflammation
- lose weight and maintain a healthy weight for life
- maintain muscle mass
- provide ample quantities of high-quality fats, proteins, and carbohydrates
- beautify your skin
- elevate your mood
- improve your brain function
- increase your energy
- improve athletic ability
- enable you to live life to the fullest

In the next part of this book, I will be recommending the foods and nutritional supplements that have a proven track record in helping us to reach these objectives. You will not only learn what they are, you will learn why and how they work, and how they can enhance your body's natural fat-reducing processes. You will also learn how your lifestyle influences your weight and health, and how you can make simple improvements that will set you on the road to weight loss, good health, and longevity.

PART II

The Three Steps

Chapter 5

STEP ONE: The 10 Top Food Groups for Permanent Weight Loss

When it is obvious that the goals cannot be reached,
don't adjust the goals, adjust the action steps.

— CONFUCIUS

I
n order for any weight-loss program to 1) work, and 2) become a lifelong lifestyle, there have to be plenty of options available. If you feel hungry or deprived, you are on the wrong program. Eating is one of the great pleasures in life, and the Perricone Weight-Loss Diet is a celebration of good food. How many weight-loss diets allow you to enjoy three meals per day and two snacks—and still lose weight? You'll never get bored (or fat) choosing from the wide variety of foods you'll find in this chapter.

In fact, I've made it easy for you. I have put my favorite foods into what I call "SuperGroups." Each SuperGroup is comprised of a different family of healthy, anti-aging, anti-inflammatory, anti-obesity choices. The food I consider to be the healthiest choice in each group is labeled "Top Choice(s)" and is followed by other healthy (and tasty) choices I call "Runners-Up."

Some of the foods in each group will be very familiar to you (especially if you've read my earlier books). Others may not be. That's why I've included information on some of the science behind each of my choices. These are all foods that will not only help you lose weight, but have proven benefits for your overall health and well-being. Feel free to mix and match foods from all these categories. Enjoy them, and enjoy the healthful benefits they provide.

FUNCTIONAL WEIGHT CONTROL FACTOR: Omega-3s
TOP CHOICE: Wild Alaskan Salmon
RUNNERS-UP: Sablefish, Sardines, Anchovies, Herring, North Atlantic Mackerel, Trout, Tuna

Everyone familiar with my previous work knows that the name "Perricone" and "salmon" are practically synonymous. In fact, as the years go by, rather than waning, I find myself becoming even more enthusiastic about this amazing food. Therefore it should come as no surprise to learn that wild salmon, the king of the superfoods, leads the pack in helping us to shed excess weight and keep it off. And the same thing that makes it such a rich, delicious, and satisfying meal—its abundance of healthful omega-3 fats—is, ironically, the same thing that makes it a top weight-control food! In chapter 4 we learned how the right fats, such as those in salmon, encourage the burning of fat for energy and discourage the storage of fat.

Top Choice: Wild Alaskan Salmon

Many Americans are unaware that wild salmon is available because of the dominance of cheaper farmed salmon in the marketplace. A number of countries and states, including Canada and California, offer wild salmon. The most abundant source of this fish is, however, Alaska. Wild salmon offers several key advantages in terms of weight control, safety, and overall health:

1. Wild and farmed salmon have comparable levels of omega-3s, but only wild salmon offers the ideal 1:2 ratio of omega-3s to omega-6s: the exact proportion that health experts recommend.

2. Wild salmon has much less cholesterol-raising, inflammation-inducing saturated fat than farmed salmon. The relatively high levels of saturated fat and omega-6 fat found in farmed salmon interfere with the benefits offered by its omega-3s.

3. Compared with wild salmon, farmed salmon is high in toxic PCBs and other

dioxin-type chemicals—the same suspected carcinogens used to poison and disfigure the democratic challenger in Ukraine's 2004 elections.

4. Only wild salmon is rich in natural astaxanthin, a uniquely potent antioxidant, anti-inflammatory nutrient. (Most farmed salmon is fed synthetic astaxanthin, which is biologically inferior to the natural form.)

5. Wild salmon offers far superior flavor and texture. It is preferred by leading chefs and restaurant chains, such as Legal Seafoods, P.F. Chang's, and many others.

6. Alaska's salmon fishery is certified as safe and sustainable by the Marine Stewardship Council and nearly all other environmental organizations, while most advise you to avoid farmed salmon. (Salmon farms pose real environmental risks.)

Runners-Up: Sardines, Anchovies, Tuna, Sablefish, and Company

All of the fish on our Runners-Up list are not only high in omega-3s, they're also safe from a mercury-and-PCBs standpoint.

◆ Sardines are a superior food because of their protein and fatty-acid content, and because their soft, edible bones add a calcium bonus to the nutritional picture.

▼

◆ Anchovies are another outstanding source of the omega-3s. Anchovies are, however, usually cured in salt. Soak them in pure water for 30 minutes before use to decrease salinity. Anchovies and sardines are also good sources of DMAE, a special nutrient that offers benefits to both the brain and the skin.

▼

◆ Tuna is another good source of omega-3s, but you need to select low-mercury types, including canned light tuna and my favorite: the young, low-weight, low-mercury Pacific albacore tuna harvested by Alaska's small-boat troller fleet. (See the Resource Guide for direct sources of fresh-frozen wild salmon, sablefish, sardines, and low-weight Pacific albacore tuna.)

▼

The Pros and Cons of Red Meat

That my personal favorite protein choice is cold-water fish—especially salmon—is no surprise. However, many of my patients and readers ask me about eating meat. Beef, pork, lamb, and veal are all excellent protein sources. As we know, protein is essential to life itself; if we do not eat adequate protein our bodies enter into an accelerated aging mode. This is because our muscles, organs, bones, cartilage, skin, and the antibodies that guard us from disease are made of protein. In fact, the very enzymes that facilitate critical chemical reactions in our body (from digestion to the building and re-building of cells) are made up of protein. As protein is digested, it is broken down into building blocks of amino acids, which are then utilized by the cells to repair themselves. Like fish and poultry, meat contains all the amino acids necessary for cellular repair.

There is a negative aspect to the consumption of red meats, and that is that they can be high in saturated fats (so can poultry—that's why we recommend that it be lean and skinless). As we have learned, too much saturated fat is inflammatory. Another negative aspect (and this includes poultry as well) is that they may also be given antibiotics, hormones, and other substances potentially harmful to humans. A European Union scientific panel has confirmed that eating beef from cattle raised on growth hormones is a potential health risk. Since 1988 the EU has had a ban on the use of such hormones and a prohibition of imported beef treated with hormones, which has led to a long-running trade disagreement with the United States and Canada. The North Americans dispute Europe's scientific evidence and allow widespread fattening of cattle with growth hormones.

If you want to eat meat, follow these safety guidelines. First, try to buy only organic meat, raised from animals that are free of antibiotics and hormones, whose feed is free of potentially dangerous chemicals—ideally the animals (including poultry) will be free-range—that is, not raised in feed lots but out in a pasture.

Another option is to consider some of the "new" types of meat being offered in the marketplace, such as bison (buffalo) and ostrich. Both have all the flavor and versatility of the red meats but present a much healthier profile, as the chart opposite attests.

♦   Perhaps the most overlooked and delicious fish on this list is SABLEFISH (aka butterfish or black cod), which, thanks to its high oil content, offers up to 58 percent more omega-3s (1.9 grams per 3.5 oz. cooked serving) than wild sockeye salmon: the kind highest in omega-3s, at 1.2 grams per 3.5 oz. serving. Its

Bison Nutrition Comparison*

Serving (3 oz.)	Calories	Protein (g)	Fat (g)	Cholesterol (mg)
Bison	85	18	2	49
Ostrich	97	22	2	58
Chicken (skinless)	140	27	3	73
Turkey (skinless)	135	25	3	59
Beef (lean, steak)	240	23	15	77
Pork (lean, loin)	275	24	19	84

* reprinted from www.mercola.com/forms/bison.htm. The bison/buffalo and ostrich that I have seen for sale have been naturally raised on organic feed. They are also competitively priced with beef, lamb, pork, and veal and are conveniently available in the meat sections of many conventional supermarkets.

smooth, luxurious texture and rich, velvety taste give sablefish a unique palate appeal much sought after by those in the know. In fact, the Japanese market buys up the vast majority of North America's Pacific sablefish catch.

So eat your wild Alaskan salmon, and take fish oil faithfully as part of a weight-reducing regimen that really works, especially if you can't or don't wish to eat fish several times a week. In addition to getting help in controlling your weight, your skin will glow with increased health and radiance!

SUPERGROUP #2: **FAVORITE FRUITS**

FUNCTIONAL WEIGHT CONTROL FACTORS: Fiber, Anti-inflammatory
Antioxidants, and other Phytonutrient Obesity-Fighters
TOP CHOICES: Apples, Pears, Grapefruit
RUNNERS-UP: All Berries, Peaches, Plums, Cherries, Pomegranates

While our Top Choices offer special advantages to the weight watcher, the vast majority of fruits are rich in anti-inflammatory antioxidants and powerful allies in preventing disease and slowing down the aging process. Most fruits share three helpful attributes.

1. **High fiber content:** Fruits are high in fiber, which moderates the impact these delightfully sweet foods would otherwise have on blood sugar levels. In addition, foods that have high fiber content give us a feeling of fullness, which helps prevent us from overeating. In fact, despite their relatively high sugar content, most fruits rank surprisingly low on the "glycemic index" and "glycemic load" scales, which measure the impact of foods on blood sugar levels.

   The moderating effect of the fiber in fruit is important because a major goal of the Perricone Weight-Loss Diet is to avoid the sharp rises in blood sugar that result in the release of insulin and, as we have learned, the storage of body fat. To make matters even worse, this "insulin overload" effect creates a vicious cycle of craving for foods (sweets, pastries, pasta, and white-flour foods) that rapidly convert to sugar in our bloodstream.

   A number of scientific studies indicate that increased fiber intake can help prevent metabolic syndrome, a deadly quartet of metabolic imbalances described in Chapter 6. And researchers at Tufts University found that people who added 14 grams of fiber to their daily diets reduced their calorie consumption by 10 percent.

2. **High phytonutrient content:** Fruits are high in anti-inflammatory, antioxidant phytonutrients–beneficial plant chemicals–many of which serve as pigments, and are concentrated in the most colorful parts, such as the peel. For example, researchers recently discovered that strawberries, blackberries, lingonberries, and

apple peels turn off key genetic switches that promote inflammation (AP-1 and NfkB). Other phytonutrients are found in the soft, white connective material called "pith" particularly prevalent in citrus fruits and concentrated right under the skin. To maximize your intake of phytonutrients, enjoy the whole fruit: pith, flesh, and peel (except citrus, pomegranate, and other obviously inedible peels). Choose organic fruits, and wash fruit well to remove any possible contaminants. (A number of fruits are waxed, another additive that you don't need. If you do get waxed fruit, remove as much of the wax as you can using a surfactant wash formulated for produce.)

3. **Sweet satisfaction:** Fruits are high in sugars (sucrose and fructose), which means that they provide quick energy to satisfy hunger. (As I've noted previously, their high levels of sugars would be a negative, pro-inflammatory influence if not for the fact that fruits are also high in fiber, which slows down the absorption of the sugars into the bloodstream.) As always, eat your protein first, and enjoy your fruits at the end of the meal to avoid any possible negative effects on blood sugar.

Top Choice: Apples

There's more than a grain of truth to the old saying "An apple a day keeps the doctor away!" Apples have landed on our list of top 10 weight-loss foods for a number of reasons:

- Apples are unusually high in fiber, with an average of 5 grams. According to the Harvard School of Public Health, we need approximately 20 to 35 grams of fiber per day, so one apple provides about 15 to 25 percent of your daily fiber requirement. Apples contain both soluble and insoluble fiber. The soluble fiber is known as "pectin," and is the substance that is added to jams and jellies to make them gel. Pectin has the power to decrease the appetite for up to four hours, making it a more effective appetite suppressant than the insoluble fiber found in grains such as wheat and rye. (Oats, like apples, are also rich in soluble fiber.)

- Despite their relatively high sugar levels, apples actually exert a stabilizing effect on blood sugar, thanks in part to their high fiber content but also because they contain phloretin: a flavonoid-type, blood-sugar-stabilizing phytonutrient found exclusively in apples. And a recent Finnish study found that eating apples can lower the risk of type 2 diabetes. The researchers attributed apples' antidiabetes effect to the antioxidant activity of quercetin, a major component of apple peels. Apple peels also appear to inhibit the growth of liver cancer and colon cancers.

▼

◆ Apples contain a wide variety of anti-inflammatory, anticancer phytonutrients, and it appears that apples may play a large role in reducing the risk of a wide variety of chronic diseases and maintaining a healthy lifestyle in general. Of the papers reviewed, apples were most consistently associated with reduced risk of cancer, heart disease, asthma, and type 2 diabetes when compared to other fruits and vegetables and other sources of flavonoids. Apple consumption was also positively associated with increased lung function and increased weight loss.

The 3 Apple-a-Day Weight Loss Secret

As we have seen, a number of studies bear out the fact that apples are a wonderful addition to any weight loss plan. However, one of my favorite stories on the role of apples in weight loss comes from an experiment conducted by Tammi Flynn, a registered dietician with a master's degree in nutrition science from Texas A&M University. Tammi, who lives in the heart of apple country in the state of Washington, came up with the concept of the "3 Apple-a-Day Plan." Her goal was to introduce more fresh produce into her clients' diets with the locally grown apples. Tammi observed that when her clients added a fresh apple to each meal, com-

pared to just eating a low-fat diet and exercise alone they had a significantly greater weight loss. Just how great she would soon find out!

Tammi, a fitness buff, was working at a local gym. She started a Get in Shape Challenge at the gym, using the plan of 3 apples per day, along with a healthy diet of low-glycemic carbohydrates, healthy fats, and quality protein. At the end of the 12-week Challenge, 346 people had lost a phenomenal 6,126 lbs. of fat (that's an average of about 18 pounds per person). And there was no question the apples played an important role in the success of the challenge.

Top Choice: Pears

Pears are actually related to apples and like that fruit have several important health benefits:

- Protection from free radicals: Pears are high in both vitamin C and copper, antioxidant nutrients that help prevent free radical damage to the cells. Both copper and vitamin C also stimulate white blood cells to fight infections and directly kill many bacteria and viruses. One medium-size pear can provide about 11 percent of the daily value your body needs for vitamin C and almost 10 percent of the copper it needs.

▼

- Promote cardiovascular and colon health: The fiber in pears has been shown to lower high cholesterol levels. It also binds to cancer-causing chemicals in the colon, preventing them from damaging colon cells.

▼

- Protection against macular degeneration: Macular degeneration is the leading cause of vision loss in older adults. A June 2004 study in the *Archives of Ophthalmology* found that eating three or more servings of fruit a day, including pears, may lower the risk of macular degeneration.

▼

- Provide vitamin B: Pears have a high concentration of folates, which make up the vitamin B-complex group. These vitamins are essential for metabolic activity and red blood cell production.

Top Choice: Grapefruit

It's back! You may or may not remember the great grapefruit diet craze of the past, which consisted mainly of a lot of grapefruit, along with a small amount of protein.

Over the years it has enjoyed intermittent popularity; however, it was finally dismissed as a fad diet with little value. But recent scientific studies are now showing that grapefruit is proving to be a worthwhile and delicious addition to the diet, especially for those who want or need to lose weight.

Grapefruit is a high-fiber, antioxidant-rich fruit that ranks low on the glycemic

Apples and Pears: A Potent Weight-Loss Pair

The authors of a study recently published in the scientific journal *Nutrition* reported that apples and pears appear to accelerate weight loss in women. Researchers from the State University in Rio de Janeiro noted that overweight women who added just 300 grams (the equivalent of three small fruits per day) to a reduced-calorie daily meal plan lost more weight than women who did not eat the fruit. In fact, the women who ate the apples or pears ended up losing 33 percent more weight than dieters getting exactly the same calories but no fruit.

The scientists have put forth several reasons as to why the addition of apples and pears to the diet might help with weight loss. One reason is that apples and pears are "low energy-density." We can actually eat more and gain greater feelings of satiety when we choose foods that are low in energy density. This is great news for all who wish to lose weight. In addition, apples and pears are rich in fiber, which enhances satiety; that is, fiber makes us feel full faster and maintains that feeling longer, thus helping prevent overeating.

[de Oliveira M, Sichieri R, Sanchez Moura A. *Nutrition* 19: 253–256, 2003; online at www.upstate.edu/nutritionjournal/]

---

scale, making it a healthy fruit to enjoy daily. (One-half of a grapefruit has only 60 calories, but a full 6 grams of fiber—more than an apple!) While the original grapefruit diet was extreme and nutritionally unbalanced, eating a grapefruit or two per day as part of a balanced diet may help you stay slim. This grapefruit-validating news comes to us from Dr. Ken Fujioka, director of Nutrition and Metabolism Research at the Scripps Clinic in San Diego, who led a study evaluating grapefruit for weight loss.

In the study, Dr. Fujioka and his colleagues assigned 100 obese men and women to one of four groups. One group received grapefruit extract, another drank grapefruit juice with each meal, the third ate half a grapefruit with each meal, while the fourth group received a placebo. Participants were asked to walk for 30 minutes three times a week.

At the end of 12 weeks the placebo group lost, on average, just less than half a pound, the extract group lost 2.4 pounds, the grapefruit juice group lost 3.3 pounds, and the fresh grapefruit group lost 3.5 pounds. The grapefruit-eating participants ate one and a half grapefruits a day, cut in half, then into four sections, separated from the skin. In this way, they were also partaking of the white pith that lines the inner skin.

Exactly how grapefruit might spur weight loss isn't known, but it appears to help insulin resistance, which develops as people become obese.

Grapefruit offers attractive health benefits. According to studies presented by the American Chemical Society at the Annual Symposium on the Potential Benefits of Citrus, grapefruit

- exhibits anti-inflammatory and antitumor properties
- reduces insulin levels and promotes weight loss
- helps ease aging-related diseases: arthritis, Alzheimer's, asthma, Parkinson's, diabetes, cataracts, and Crohn's disease

Both red and pink grapefruit are members of a special group of fruits that contain lycopene, an open-chain unsaturated carotenoid that gives that vibrant red color to tomatoes, blood oranges, guava, rosehips, and watermelon. Research indicates that lycopene has a protective effect against heart disease, certain cancers, and macular degeneration, a leading cause of blindness.

One note, however. Grapefruit has been shown to have negative interactions with some commonly prescribed medications. Apparently the flavonoid compounds in grapefruit juice inhibit a special enzyme in the intestines that is responsible for the breakdown and absorption of many medications, including antihistamines and statins (the drugs prescribed for lowering cholesterol). If you take these or any medications, check with your doctor before adding grapefruit to your diet.

Runners-Up: Berries, Peaches, Plums, Cherries

I chose these fruits as runners-up for several reasons. Each of these fruits, especially the berries, is very high in anti-inflammatory antioxidants. And while all of them taste quite sweet, they rank as moderate on the glycemic index and glycemic load scales, and will therefore not raise blood sugar too high or too rapidly.

Berries are one of Nature's very finest antioxidant foods and blueberries top the list. They're loaded with a variety of phytonutrients, including anthocyanins, which give them their rich blue color. Just one-half cup of blueberries per day will double

Luo Han Kuo (LHK) — World's Most Powerful Antioxidant?

We know that many fruits are powerful antioxidants, but here's one you may never have heard of: Luo Han Kuo (LHK). This Chinese fruit has been recognized and prized as a food and medicinal herb for use in Traditional Chinese Medicine (TCM) for more than 1,000 years. The Chinese have long referred to LHK as the "fruit of longevity."

This rare fruit grows only in the unique microclimate found in the mountains of Guangxi Province, China, home to the only known place on earth where the number of people over 100 years old actually increased in 2004.

Use of this "magic fruit" has been the same for more than a thousand years: LHK cleanses and nourishes the lungs, promotes general respiratory health, and enhances overall immune functions. Modern research demonstrates the importance of antioxidants in respiratory health.

Although Luo Han Kuo is a fruit, it is sold in the U.S. as a dietary supplement in small packets and can be used like a tea; one packet is mixed with hot or cold water. LHK is an indispensable therapeutic agent that can be used every day.

your antioxidant intake—even if you already eat a diet with plenty of fresh fruits and vegetables. In fact, you could greatly accelerate your entire anti-inflammatory regimen by including daily intake of two foods: blueberries and broccoli sprouts (more about them in SuperGroup #10).

Blueberries actually help reverse the decline in brain function and impaired balance, two symptoms often seen in older people. They also prevent the death of our cells while increasing our ability to release dopamine. A stimulating, energizing neurotransmitter, dopamine increases brain energy production while maintaining youthful brain function.

Berries are an ideal and delicious anti-inflammatory alternative to sweets. That said, both fruits and vegetables are an indispensable part of a healthy diet and a real plus to anyone wanting to lose weight. In fact, there are numerous studies that show that by incorporating fruits and vegetables into your diet, you can *actually change* your body mass index and waist circumference.

SUPERGROUP #3: FATS FROM FRUITS TO FIGHT BODY FAT

FUNCTIONAL WEIGHT CONTROL FACTORS: Anti-inflammatory Antioxidants, Monounsaturated Fats
TOP CHOICES: Avocado, Açaí, Olives
RUNNER-UP: Coconut

We don't normally think of a fruit as a source of dietary fats. However, there are a few delightfully delicious and nutritious exceptions to the rule. Avocados, açaí, olives, and coconut are fruits that are rich sources of monounsaturated fats (MUFAs). These special types of fats help prevent many diseases, help us absorb nutrients from our plant foods, nourish our skin, and help provide that all-important feeling of satiety.

Top Choice: Avocado

Although we think of the avocado as a vegetable, it is actually a fruit–and a delicious one at that. For years many people avoided avocados because they are high in fat. However, most of the fat in an avocado is monounsaturated, the kind believed by some scientists to protect against heart disease and certain cancers. In addition, monounsaturated fat is burned more efficiently after exercise than saturated fat, a fact that may significantly contribute to long-term weight loss. A study from Brigham and Women's Hospital in Boston showed that diets high in monounsaturated fat like that found in avocados can be more effective than low-fat plans for weight loss and maintenance.

Avocados also contain omega-3 fatty acids, which, as we know, facilitate weight loss, are beneficial for heart health, and reduce inflammation. Creamy, buttery avocados make an excellent substitute for foods high in inflammatory saturated fats such as butter, cream cheese, and sour cream.

Avocados are cholesterol-free, sodium-free, and low in saturated fat. They're a nutrient-dense food that offers potassium, magnesium, folate, dietary fiber, riboflavin, and vitamins C, E, and B$_6$. They are also rich in anti-inflammatory, antiaging, disease-fighting phytochemicals including lutein and other antioxidants.

Research shows that, ounce for ounce, avocados rank highest among the 20 most frequently consumed fruits in the following phytochemicals and nutrients:

◆ Lutein–may protect against prostate cancer and eye disease such as cataracts and macular degeneration.

▼

◆ Vitamin E–a powerful antioxidant known to slow the aging process and protect against heart disease and various forms of cancer.

▼

◆ Glutathione–functions as an antioxidant like vitamin E to neutralize free radicals that can cause cell damage and lead to disease.

▼

◆ Beta-sitosterol–lowers blood cholesterol levels. Avocados contain four times as much beta-sitosterol as oranges, previously reported as the highest fruit source of this phytochemical.

▼

◆ Folate–promotes healthy cell and tissue development. Folate is especially important for women of childbearing age as it helps protect against birth defects.

▼

◆ Potassium–helps balance the body's electrolytes. Avocados contain 60 percent more potassium than bananas.

▼

◆ Magnesium–helps produce energy and is important for muscle contraction and relaxation.

▼

◆ Fiber–lowers cholesterol and reduces risk of heart attack.

Current research has shown avocados to be particularly helpful and healthful in a variety of ways:

◆ *Diabetes Prevention:* Recent guidelines issued by the American Diabetes Association emphasize a diet rich in monounsaturated fats–such as is found in avocados–to raise good cholesterol levels and promote blood sugar regulation. In its most recent position statement on dietary recommendations for the prevention and treatment of diabetes, the American Diabetes Association states that diets high in monounsaturated fatty acids improve glucose tolerance and lipid (fat) levels compared with diets high in saturated fat. Furthermore, diets enriched with MUFAs may also reduce insulin resistance.

[Franz MJ, et al. Evidence-based Nutrition Principles and Recommendations for the Treatment and Prevention of Diabetes and Related Complications (Technical Review). *Diabetes Care* 2002;25:148–198.]

▼

◆ *Fitness:* Active individuals who work out 30 minutes a day can stay energized by consuming monounsaturated fat, as found in avocados, because monounsaturated fats burn efficiently and provide stamina for a workout. Researchers at the University of Wisconsin found that women who ate healthy monounsaturated fat before a cycling workout burned fat more efficiently. Approximately 50 percent of the fat was burned after heavy exercise, 39 percent after light exercise, and 34 percent after resting. [Votruba SB, Atkinson RL, Schoeller DA. Prior exercise increases dietary oleate, but not palmitate oxidation. *Obesity Research* 2003;11(12):1509–1518.]

▼

◆ *Obesity/Weight Management:* Eating foods with a low energy density, such as avocados, can support a healthy body weight because they make you feel satisfied with fewer calories. Energy density is the amount of calories in a portion of food. Because of their high water and fiber content avocados are considered a low energy-dense food–few calories per ounce. By filling up on foods with a low energy density, satiety is achieved with fewer calories and they can help maintain a healthy weight. You don't need to eat an entire avocado to reap the benefits; one-fifth of an avocado contains only 55 calories. [Rolls, Barbara and Barnett, Robert A. *The Volumetrics Weight-Control Plan,* Harper Torch, New York 2003.] And researchers at Pennsylvania State University found that lean and obese women who consumed foods with a low energy density consumed fewer calories than when they ate foods with higher energy density. [Bell EA, Rolls BJ. Energy density of foods affects energy intake across multiple levels of fat content in lean and obese women. *Am J Clin Nutr* 2001;73(6):1010–1018.]

To learn more health and nutrition facts and enjoy delicious recipes, visit www.avocado.org.

Top Choice: Açaí

I first introduced açaí in *The Perricone Promise* as one of the top ten superfoods for anti-aging and overall health. Because of its excellent fatty acid, amino acid, and anti-inflammatory profile, it also deserves star billing in the Perricone Weight-Loss Diet. One of the qualities I most love about açaí is that it provides us with quality protein, healthy fat, and powerful antioxidants all in one amazing berry. Açaí pulp contains:

- ◆ A remarkable concentration of antioxidants that help combat premature aging, with 10 times more antioxidants than red grapes and 10–30 times the anthocyanins of red wine.

▼

- ◆ A synergy of monounsaturated (healthy) fats, dietary fiber, and phytosterols, to help promote cardiovascular system and digestive tract health.

▼

- ◆ An almost perfect essential amino acid complex in conjunction with valuable trace minerals, vital to proper muscle contraction and regeneration.

Açaí is good for weight loss because it contains cyanidin, a highly antioxidant phytochemical compound. Japanese researchers have discovered that cyanidin may have the effect of draining body fat as well as reducing fat absorption.

A Note About Phytosterols

Phytosterols are plant compounds that are chemically similar to cholesterol. However, unlike ingested cholesterol, which is derived from animal sources (and when eaten, raises our cholesterol levels), phytosterols do just the opposite. They block dietary cholesterol from being absorbed into the bloodstream, which can lower cholesterol levels. Some phytosterols stimulate insulin secretion, which may help control blood sugar. In addition, phytosterols help prevent heart disease and have anti-inflammatory properties, helping to reduce inflammation in arthritis and other autoimmune diseases.

Açaí is also rich in monounsaturated oleic acid, which is the chief fatty acid found in olive oil. One of the outstanding benefits of oleic acid is its ability to help the omega-3 fish oils penetrate the cell membrane. The combination of these two fatty acids helps to maintain flexible and supple cell membranes. This allows all hormones, neurotransmitters, and insulin receptors to function more efficiently; critically important to maintain homeostasis, that is, keeping the body working as it should because all of its systems are in balance. Only then can we lose weight and prevent unwanted weight gain.

Top Choice: Olives (and Extra Virgin Olive Oil)

Long prized for its robust and delicious taste, extra virgin olive oil has also gained fame as the cornerstone of the famous Mediterranean diet. Researchers have consistently found that in countries such as Spain, Greece, Italy, and France, where people most closely follow the traditional diets of their ancestors, inhabitants not only live longer, they have decreased incidence of heart disease, cancer, and other degenerative diseases.

One of the most important constituents of olive oil is oleic acid, which is vital in keeping the outer portion of the cell, known as the cell plasma membrane, supple, thereby allowing nutrients to enter the cell and wastes to exit.

Hardly a day goes by without a new discovery of the benefits of olive oil and its constituents. Dr. Javier Menendez of Northwestern University's Feinberg School of Medicine in Chicago, found that oleic acid blocks the action of a cancer-causing oncogene called HER-2/neu, which is found in about 30 percent of breast cancer patients.

Olive oil can also be an important part of a weight-loss plan. Experience shows that there is less obesity among the Mediterranean people, who consume the most olive oil. (Don't forget that they also consume large amounts of omega-3 fatty acids in the form of fish, including anchovies and sardines.) It has also been demonstrated that an olive-oil-rich diet leads to greater and longer-lasting weight loss than a low-calorie diet. And, because of its delicious taste, it acts as a great stimulus to eat our vegetables! Researchers have also found that a diet rich in extra virgin olive oil can actually assist in the redistribution of fat, helping to eliminate the dangerous visceral fat around the midsection.

According to the International Olive Oil Council (www.iooc.com), an olive-oil-rich diet may also help to prevent or delay the onset of diabetes. It does so by preventing insulin resistance and its possible pernicious implications by raising HDL cholesterol, lowering triglycerides, and ensuring better blood sugar level control and lower blood pressure. It has been demonstrated that a diet rich in olive oil, low in saturated fats, moderately rich in low-glycemic carbohydrates and soluble fiber from fruit, vegetables, legumes, and whole grains such as whole oats or old-fashioned oatmeal is the most effective approach for diabetics. Besides lowering the "bad" low-density lipoproteins, this type of diet improves blood sugar control and enhances insulin sensitivity. These benefits have been documented in both childhood and adult diabetes.

Runner-Up: Coconuts (and Coconut Oil)

If your only knowledge of coconuts comes from the Marx Brothers' classic film or a few piña coladas sipped in a tropical paradise, visit www.spectrumorganics.com and learn the good news! Long vilified as an unhealthy food choice, coconuts and coconut oil are now rightly taking their place as not only a healthy food and a healthy type of fat, but also as a food that appears to promote weight loss. According to the study "Medium-Chain Triglycerides Increase Energy Expenditure and Decrease Adiposity in Overweight Men," published in the medical journal *Obesity Research,* diets rich in coconut potentially stimulate weight loss by increasing metabolism, and may be considered aids in the prevention of obesity.

Coconut contains saturated fat. In general, I recommend you stay away from these fats, found often in most fried foods, full-fat dairy products, and meat (see Chapter 4). However, saturated fats appear both in animal foods and plant foods. Most of what we consume in the United States consists of artery-clogging, "long-chain" saturated fats derived from animals. But the plant-based medium-chain fatty acids (or medium-chain triglycerides [MCT], as they are known in scientific circles) tend to digest quickly, producing energy and stimulating the metabolism—the reason oils like coconut are popular with athletes. A number of studies have found that the medium-chain triglycerides in coconut oil are not readily converted into stored fats nor can they be readily used by the body to make larger fat molecules.

It is studies such as these, along with one that showed conclusively that coconut oil actually increased metabolism after a meal, that have given coconut oil its reputation as a weight-loss magic bullet. While I find this an extreme claim, I do feel that there is good science showing that by replacing unhealthy or less healthy fats such as butter, margarine, and conventional vegetable oils with coconut oil we will store less fat and increase our metabolism. Coconut oil is practically tasteless, which means that it will not adversely affect flavors of food.

Coconut oil also offers additional health benefits and has been shown to have antiviral and antimicrobial properties due to the lauric acid fraction in the oil. Its fatty-acid profile consists primarily of caprylic and lauric acids, which support immune function. Coconut oil is also used medicinally for candida and yeast infections. Its healing reputation is attributed to the caproic fatty acids found in high concentrations compared to other plant material.

One final note on coconut. Tender coconut water appears to be a really outstanding beverage. Long revered for rehydration and as a health and beauty aid in tropical regions around the world, it is only now being introduced to the rest of us. It not only stimulates metabolism, it provides many other benefits. Since it is low in calories and has a natural balance of sodium, potassium, calcium, and magnesium, it makes a healthy electrolyte drink. It has also been shown to have antiviral, antifungal, and antimicrobial properties. It helps to heal damage induced by antibiotics and toxins in the digestive tract, it boosts poor circulation, it balances pH, and it may even help prevent cancer.

SUPERGROUP #4: SPICE THINGS UP TO KEEP WEIGHT DOWN

FUNCTIONAL WEIGHT CONTROL FACTORS: Anti-inflammatory Antioxidants, and other Phytonutrient Obesity-Fighters
TOP CHOICE: Cinnamon
RUNNERS-UP: Turmeric, Fenugreek, Cloves, Allspice, Nutmeg, Bay Leaf

The best way to avoid the vicious boom-and-bust blood sugar cycle is to limit intake of high-glycemic carbohydrates and increase your intake of supplements (such as chromium) and foods proven to help stabilize blood sugar—especially beans, nuts, seeds, healthful proteins, all members of the onion family (including garlic), and green vegetables. New studies now indicate that we can add fragrant spices like cinnamon, fenugreek, cloves, and turmeric to the list.

Top Choice: Cinnamon

The USDA Human Nutrition Research Center in Beltsville, Maryland, is a world leader in research on links between nutrition and disease. When their scientists conducted a recent study, they were amazed to discover that the blood sugar levels of volunteers who ate apple pie didn't rise, as would be expected in response to a food that is high in sugar and refined flour.

The scientists at the USDA soon determined that one ingredient in their apple pie—cinnamon—was responsible for keeping blood sugar levels on an even keel. That said, avoid apple pie if you want to stay slim and healthy—eat the apple and sprinkle a little cinnamon on it! They later determined that the phytonutrient compounds responsible for cinnamon's beneficial effect on blood sugar control—flavon-3-ol polyphenol-class antioxidants—are similar to those found in grapes, berries, cocoa, and green tea.

Flavon-3-ol antioxidants enhance the stabilizing effect of insulin on blood sugar and decrease insulin resistance in two ways. First, these antioxidants activate enzymes that stimulate insulin receptors. Remember that when we are insulin resistant our cells cannot sense the presence of insulin. By sensitizing these receptors we are potentiating insulin's power to reduce blood sugar levels. Second, they enhance the effects of insulin-signaling pathways within skeletal muscle tissue.

Because the flavon-3-ol antioxidants in cinnamon increase insulin sensitivity, they help the body to lessen the harmful effects of high-glycemic carbohydrates, which include the up and down blood sugar cycle that causes cravings for dietary carbs, and the chronic inflammation that promotes obesity. Because flavon-3-ol antioxidants enhance insulin sensitivity, more of your blood glucose enters the cells where it belongs and blood sugar levels stabilize, effectively quenching the inflammation and ending carbohydrate craving.

One of the researchers on the USDA team, Alam Khan, went on to test cinnamon in a placebo-controlled clinical trial. Sixty volunteers with type 2 diabetes were divided into groups. Half received a placebo, while the remainder were divided into three groups that took different doses of cinnamon in capsule form–doses equivalent to ¼, ½, or 1¾ teaspoon–for 20 days, following meals.

As hoped, postprandial (after-meal) blood sugar levels decreased sharply–by 23 to 30 percent–among the participants who received cinnamon, while there were no significant changes in the placebo-capsule group. And the researchers were delighted to discover that all of the cinnamon-capsule groups also experienced very substantial reductions in their blood levels of triglycerides (23 to 30 percent) and total cholesterol (13 to 26 percent), while the two highest dose groups also enjoyed a 10 to 24 percent reduction in levels of LDL (bad) cholesterol.

The cinnamon surprises kept coming. Three weeks after the study ended, the groups that had received cinnamon continued to enjoy healthier blood sugar levels, an unexpected result meaning that cinnamon works its metabolic magic even if you don't eat it every day. For reasons that remain unclear, the group that took the lowest dose of cinnamon enjoyed the most durable improvement in blood sugar control.

The USDA also reported that the active components of cinnamon are found in the water-soluble portion of cinnamon and are not present in cinnamon oil, which is largely fat-soluble. In addition to ground cinnamon consumed directly, one can also make a cinnamon tea and let the solids settle to the bottom or use cinnamon sticks, which make for a nice clear tea. Cinnamon can also be added to oatmeal, salads, meats, curries, soups, and stews, because the active components are not destroyed by heat.

They further found that consuming roughly one-half teaspoon or less of cinnamon per day leads to the aforementioned dramatic improvements in blood sugar, cholesterol, LDL cholesterol, and triglycerides. Intake of cinnamon at these levels is very safe and there should not be any side effects. However, cinnamon can also act as a blood thinner. If you are taking any prescription drug or are being treated for any health condition, consult with your primary physician before making any alterations to your current dietary plan.

Runners-Up: Turmeric, Fenugreek, Cloves, and Company

When the USDA tested 49 herbs, spices, and medicinal plants for their insulin-enhancing activity, cinnamon ranked number one. The closest runners-up were turmeric and fenugreek, followed by cloves, allspice, nutmeg, and bay leaves.

◆ The results of a pair of animal studies suggest that **turmeric**–one of the polyphenol-rich SuperFoods I first discussed in *The Perricone Promise*–may also be of use in the fight against elevated blood sugar. Curcumin, one of the active constituents in turmeric, has both antioxidant and anti-inflammatory properties and has been shown to reduce Alzheimer's-related inflammation in the brain tissue. It also aids digestion, helps fight infection, and guards against heart attacks. Turmeric is an indispensable ingredient of curry, whose many fragrant herbs and spices deliver outstanding antioxidant, anti-inflammatory benefits.

▼

◆ Another Indian culinary standby–**fenugreek**–may offer significant blood sugar stabilizing effects. Fenugreek seed contains fibrous compounds that slow digestion. As a result, any sugars and high-glycemic starches occurring in foods get absorbed more slowly, which prevents blood sugar levels from rising as fast as they otherwise would. Fenugreek also contains a unique amino acid called 4-hydroxyisoleucine, which, in diabetics, improves blood sugar control and decreases insulin resistance. This amino acid may also promote storage of dietary carbohydrates as glycogen, rather than as hard-to-lose body fat.

FUNCTIONAL WEIGHT CONTROL FACTORS: Anti-inflammatory Antioxidants, Fiber, and Phytonutrient Obesity-Fighters
TOP CHOICE: Chili Peppers
RUNNERS-UP: Cayenne, Chili Powder, Red Pepper Flakes

Hot chili peppers are rich in powerful anti-inflammatory antioxidants (carotenoids and flavonols), as are salsas and curries containing chilies and other tropical spices. But chili peppers deserve a place of spicy distinction, because they offer unique weight control attributes.

The native cuisines of many hot countries are chock full of spicy chilies, even though eating them tends to raise body temperature, a seeming disadvantage in a steamy climate. However, chilies also make people sweat, which lowers body temperature. In other words, chilies may help people feel cooler in the long run, by acting as culinary "air conditioners."

The spicy constituents of chili peppers are phytonutrient compounds called capsaicinoids. One of these—capsaicin—is the most abundant and beneficial capsaicinoid in chilies. Capsaicin exerts strong anti-inflammatory effects and possesses proven anti-cancer and heart-health properties. Capsaicin is also a potent topical analgesic that relieves pain by inhibiting production of a neuropeptide called "substance P" (SP). A great way to up your hot pepper intake is to add salsa to eggs, cottage cheese, grilled fish and poultry, and other fundamentally bland foods. A healthy dash of Tabasco® sauce will also do the trick and liven up soups, salads, sauces, stews, and a wide variety of savory dishes.

There are four ways that capsaicin aids weight control:

1. Suppresses the appetite.

2. Raises your metabolic rate temporarily, which stimulates your body to release adrenaline, thus increasing your body's propensity to burn stored body fat and sugars (glycogen).

3. Stimulates thermogenesis. Therefore, it comes as no surprise that capsaicin is a key constituent in many of the most popular diet supplements, a turn of events prompted in part by the FDA's banning of ephedra—perhaps the most effective thermogenic agent—because of the risks it poses to people with heart conditions. In sharp contrast to ephedra, capsaicin is actively heart-healthy.

4. Inhibits spikes in blood sugar for about 30 minutes after it is ingested, thereby reducing the risk of an insulin response.

Thanks to a Japanese-Canadian research team that has conducted several studies on the subject, it is clear that capsaicin tends to reduce the amount of calories consumed at a meal. Their most recent study, published in 2004, was designed to determine whether capsaicin's consumption-cutting effect is linked to the "hot" sensations it produces in the mouth or is purely physiological in nature. This study also showed that it takes a hefty, relatively "hot" dose of capsaicin to reduce calorie consumption at a meal.

Thankfully for folks who are not fond of spicy hot food, the study's findings indicate that calorie consumption is reduced by capsaicin, whether it is added to food or swallowed in capsule form with a meal. That's good news for every diner: those who do not enjoy hot, spicy foods can just pop a capsaicin pill as they begin a meal, and those who like to "feel the burn" will be even more eager to let loose with the hot sauce!

Top Choice: Chili Peppers (and Hot Chili Sauces)

While any source of capsaicin—dried or fresh—will do the consumption-cutting trick, I prefer whole chilies (fresh or canned). My preference stems from the fact that in addition to capsaicinoids and vitamin C, whole chilies contain the widest possible range of anti-inflammatory, antioxidant phytonutrients in the highest possible concentrations. The predominant phytonutrients in chilies are colorless flavonols (especially quercetin) and colorful anthocyanins (purple peppers) and carotenoids (beta-carotene and capsanthin).

If you can't take their full heat, you can reduce the hotness by removing some or all of the seeds before cooking. Just remember that the "hotter" you make the meal—that is, the more capsaicin it contains—the greater will be its appetite-suppressing effect.

Runners-Up: Red Pepper or Crushed Red Pepper (Red Pepper Flakes)

Dried chilies, in the form of red pepper powders or flakes, offer a convenient way to get the consumption-cutting power of capsaicin while spicing up your cuisine. They lack the full range of phytonutrients found in fresh or canned chilies, but still constitute a healthful, capsaicin-rich complement to meals.

"Red pepper" is the generic name for all powdered chili products. Among red peppers, cayenne pepper powder packs the hottest punch. "Crushed red pepper" and "red pepper flakes" are interchangeable terms that refer to a blend of red flakes of dried chili and dried yellow chili seeds. Manufacturers may employ a variety of chilies to make crushed red pepper, although ancho chilies are the most common.

The relative hotness of chilies is expressed in Scoville heat units, which reflects the amount of capsaicin in parts per million. Accordingly, one part per million of capsaicin is expressed as 15 Scoville units. Sweet bell peppers are the baseline, at zero Scoville units, while habañero peppers rank near the top of the scale, at a searing 250,000 Scoville units. The more mature the pepper, the redder and hotter it will be, so a red jalapeño will be hotter than a green one. (Like bell peppers, chili peppers start out green and turn yellow-red-orange as they mature.)

Experiment to find your favorite chilies: these brief descriptions will give you some guidance (see the Resource Guide for more chili information).

◆ Anaheim chilies range from mild to moderately hot and are sold in both the green and red stages of development. The strands of red chilies found in stores—called ristras—are usually made with mature red Anaheims. The classic Mexican chiles rellenos, or stuffed chiles, are also made with Anaheims. Scoville units: 1,000–1,500.

▼

◆ Ancho is the term applied to dried poblano peppers (dark red to brown-black in color), but is sometimes erroneously used to label fresh poblanos. Like fresh poblanos, ancho chilies range from mild to moderately hot. Scoville units: 1,000–1,500.

▼

◆ Cayenne peppers rank among the hotter chilies and are most often sold as a ground, dried powder. Scoville units: 30,000–50,000.

- Chipotle peppers are simply smoked jalapeños and form the basis of canned adobo sauce. Scoville units: 2,500–10,000.

- Habañeros—also called Scotch bonnets—are small yellow-orange, lantern-shaped peppers. The hotness of habañero peppers is surpassed by only a few rare Asian varieties, and it can take a little while to manifest fully, so wait before taking a second bite of habañero-spiced food. Also, be forewarned. These peppers truly are lethally hot, so even if you think your "hot" threshold is high, use extreme caution when eating or even handling these peppers. Scoville units: 80,000–300,000.

- Jalapeño peppers vary widely in hotness, sometimes very mild, and sometimes quite hot, with the difference immediately apparent. Jalapeño peppers are usually sold at the dark green stage, but fully ripe red jalapeños can also be found. Scoville units: 2,500–5,000.

- Poblano peppers range from mild to hot, and are often used—roasted and peeled—in recipes, or stuffed to make chiles rellenos. Scoville units: 1,000–1,500.

- Serrano chilies are very hot peppers popular in Mexico and the U.S. Southwest, where they are used primarily in salsas, usually in their green stage. Scoville units: 10,000–23,000.

As mentioned, be careful when handling chili peppers. Wash your hands immediately after touching their interior parts—especially the light-colored veins, the walls, and the seeds, as this is the source of their capsaicin. Don't wait to wash, lest you forget and touch your eyes or sensitive skin areas absentmindedly! In fact, it's smart to handle chilies with rubber gloves.

If you want to reduce their hotness, cut chilies open and remove the seeds and ribs. To further reduce their hotness, soak the peppers in cool salted water for an hour.

SUPERGROUP #6: SEEDS AND NUTS TO FILL YOU UP

FUNCTIONAL WEIGHT CONTROL FACTORS: Anti-inflammatory Antioxidants, Essential Fats, Protein, Fiber, Lignans
TOP CHOICES: Sesame Seeds, Flaxseeds
RUNNERS-UP: Almonds, Walnuts, Hazelnuts, Sunflower Seeds, Pumpkin Seeds

Adding nuts and seeds to your daily diet will provide the following benefits. They

◆ decrease your risk of cancer, heart disease, and diabetes
◆ help control weight with no hunger pangs
◆ reduce the visible signs of aging such as wrinkles and sagging skin

Nuts are high in protein and also in "healthy" fats. Because of this, a small handful of nuts will provide satiety for hours, helping you to eliminate hunger pangs and food cravings. Traditionally we thought that a healthy snack for weight loss was carrot sticks, or celery stalks, or apple slices—and we all know the level of satiety those foods provide—practically zero when eaten alone, unaccompanied by a source of healthy fat and protein. However, when we add a few nuts to the equation, or spread a teaspoon of fresh almond butter or tahini on the celery stalk or apple slice, a very different picture begins to emerge. Our hunger is satisfied and our energy level is maintained. The fat in the nuts or nut butter also facilitates the absorption of the vital phytonutrients, vitamins, minerals, and anti-inflammatory antioxidants found in the fruits and vegetables. So don't be afraid to enjoy a handful of nuts or seeds as a stand-alone snack, in salads, or in stir-fries. Just use moderation and keep servings limited to the aforementioned small handful per serving.

Top Choice: Sesame Seeds

New research has placed the tiny **sesame seed** on the top of the nut and seed pyramid when it comes to promoting healthy weight loss.

While sesame seeds (*Sesamum indicum*) are one of the world's oldest cultivated foods, they can now take honors as one of the world's newest weight-loss wonders! Sesame seeds and its lignans (sesamin, sesamolin, sesamolinol–phytonutrients that have powerful antioxidant, antifungal, antibacterial, antiviral, and anticarcinogenic properties) offer many health benefits including:

- lower cholesterol
- act as an anti-inflammatory
- increase levels of antioxidants
- prevent high blood pressure
- increase levels of vitamin E
- contain three times as much calcium as an equivalent amount of milk
- are rich in magnesium, an important mineral for maintaining the nervous system
- protect the liver from oxidative damage
- promote fat burning
- work in concert with important nutrients including gamma tocopherol, conjugated linoleic acid (CLA), and fish oil to increase the power and bioavailability of these substances
- stimulators of fatty-acid oxidation, one of the key processes involved in weight control
- when combined with fish oil, sesame helps to enhance the fish oil's anti-inflammatory effects by protecting it from lipid peroxidation (the process by which fatty acids get oxidized)

According to an outstanding and thoroughly researched article published on the Life Extension website (www.lef.org), many studies indicate that the lignans found in sesame may actually increase the oxidation of fatty acids in the liver. Scientists believe that if we can maximize the liver's oxidation of fatty acids, this will encourage the loss of fat. When animal studies were conducted in which rats were given the sesame lignan sesamin, there was a significant increase in the activity of many fatty-acid oxidation enzymes. This activity was accelerated in rats that were also given fish oil in conjunction with the sesamin. In another study, the addition of sesamin to conjugated linoleic acid (CLA), a fatty acid known to promote weight loss, promoted even greater weight loss, as measured by a reduction in adipose tissue weight. Sesame lignans thus appear to have a synergistic effect, enhancing the benefits of fish oil and CLA in promoting optimal fat burning and healthy weight.

Unfortunately for many of us, the only time we have ever even seen a sesame seed has been on the top of the bun of our Big Mac®. An easy way to enjoy sesame seeds is by eating hummus (a staple in Middle Eastern cuisine), which is often seasoned with tahini, a rich, creamy sauce made of ground sesame seeds. With this amazing array of health and weight-loss benefits, perhaps now this ancient seed can take its rightful place in our modern diets.

Top Choice: Flaxseeds

Flaxseeds are a delicious and very nutritious addition to many meals. Flaxseed contains

- large amounts of omega-3 fatty acid and alpha linolenic acid (ALA), an essential fatty acid that our bodies can't make from other foods
- very high amounts of dietary fiber, both soluble and insoluble
- lignans that have apparent anticarcinogenic action
- nutrients including proteins, carbohydrates, and minerals
- a high concentration of potassium*

According to the U.S. Department of Agriculture, flaxseed contains 27 identifiable cancer-preventive compounds. Medical sources abound that have published clinical results concluding that flax can have a positive impact on your overall health and can be helpful with

- cancer
- weight loss
- heart disease
- diabetes
- hypertension

Other properties of a diet rich in flax as compiled by the North Dakota State University Department of Plant Sciences include:

*North Dakota State University Department of Plant Sciences

- reduction of LDL cholesterol and triglycerides
- anti-inflammatory effects
- natural laxative effects of dietary fiber
- helps glucose control in diabetics
- softens skin and improves coat (fur) of animals
- reduces some psoriasis in people and other animals
- ameliorates renal disease (lupus nephritis) with favorable effects on plasma lipids and blood pressure

To experience the benefits of flax, consume between 3 and 6 tablespoons of flaxseeds per day. Always buy organic flaxseed and grind fresh in a coffee grinder for optimum benefits. Store in the freezer. You may also take organic cold-pressed flax oil. Buy in small quantities and keep refrigerated to protect it from rancidity—an ever-present hazard with all nuts, seeds, and their oils.

Runners-Up: Almonds, Walnuts, Hazelnuts, Sunflower Seeds, Pumpkin Seeds

For optimal health, enjoy a variety of nuts and seeds daily, especially:

- Almonds: High in riboflavin, copper, magnesium, and vitamin E, only a quarter of a cup provides 4 grams of fiber. They are also a very good source of calcium.

- Walnuts: A good source of linolenic acid, which can be converted into omega-3 fatty acids in the body. Walnuts are also high in copper and manganese.

- Hazelnuts: These nuts contain nearly 91 percent monounsaturated fat and less than 4 percent saturated fat. More than 30 tree-nut studies indicate this high level of monounsaturated fat is likely responsible for a reduction in both total blood and LDL cholesterol levels when hazelnuts are consumed as part of a low saturated fat diet. Hazelnuts also contain significant amounts of protein, fiber, iron, phosphorus, vitamins B_1, B_2, C, and E, folate, and many other essential nutrients.

- Sunflower seeds: An excellent source of vitamin E for neutralizing free radicals and lowering the risk of cardiovascular disease. Sunflower seeds are also a good source of magnesium, which is essential for healthy bones, to help lower blood pressure and prevent migraine headaches. These seeds also contain selenium, a trace mineral that has been shown to inhibit the proliferation of cancer cells.

▼

◆ Pumpkin seeds: Pumpkin seeds contain chemicals called cucurbitacins that help prevent the body from converting testosterone into a more potent form of the hormone called dihydrotestosterone. Inhibiting that conversion reduces the production of prostate cells, thereby reducing the enlargement of the prostate. Pumpkin seeds also contain zinc, which helps keep skin clear and prevent osteoporosis.

SUPERGROUP #7: BEANS AND LENTILS (LEGUME FAMILY) FOR STABILIZING BLOOD SUGAR

FUNCTIONAL WEIGHT CONTROL FACTORS: Fiber, Resistant Starch, Starch Blockers, and Phytonutrient Obesity-Fighters

TOP CHOICES: Dried Beans, including Kidney, Pinto, Navy, Red, and Black Beans, Lentils, Chickpeas, Mung Beans

RUNNERS-UP: All are recommended

Believe it or not, there is one "starchy" food group that provides total satiety, satisfies energy and protein needs, delivers anti-inflammatory, antioxidant phytonutrients, burns body fat, and moderates blood levels of both blood sugar and insulin! That food group is legumes–dried beans, lentils, and company. These humble, unassuming (and inexpensive) dietary mainstays are prized by both traditional cultures and contemporary fans of ethnic cuisines. Not only are they supremely satisfying, providing that much missed feeling of "fullness" dieters long for, beans also serve double duty as ace weight-control allies. The evidence is crystal clear: beans prompt more burning of body fat, stabilize blood sugar more strongly, and pack much more protein than any other plant food family.

A meal with legumes raises blood sugar very slowly and moderately, and even moderates the blood sugar response to the next meal you eat, whether this next meal includes beans or not. And beans exert their beneficial effects when mixed with relatively high-glycemic foods (sugars, refined flour products) yet still wield a potent stabilizing influence on blood sugar levels and subsequent insulin levels.

Beans owe most of their weight-control clout to four factors:

1. *Fiber:* The nondigestible starches we call fiber–in which beans are especially rich–are filling, providing feelings of satiety from even small amounts, while also stabilizing blood sugar: two key weight-control enhancers. A great number of population studies show that, after adjusting for all other factors, higher fiber intake is associated with lower body weight, less body fat, and lower body mass index (weight-to-height ratio). Results from clinical trials are more mixed, although in most cases, when people had higher fiber intake there was a decrease in their overall food consumption and a subsequent drop in their body weight.

2. *Resistant starch (RS):* These fiberlike carbohydrates are the unsung heroes of weight control. They increase the rate at which the body burns (oxidizes) body fat, do not cause unhealthy spikes in blood sugar levels, and prevent other, higher glycemic foods in a meal from doing so.

As its name implies, resistant starch *resists* digestion and absorption as it passes through the small intestine, where most dietary starch gets digested. It then passes into the large intestine where it behaves much like insoluble fiber, promoting the growth of beneficial bacteria and the production of disease-preventive fatty acids.

Unlike a true fiber, some portion of dietary RS eventually gets digested, but it happens much too slowly to produce an inflammatory spike in blood sugar levels. Better yet, when you eat a small amount of RS—for instance, a handful of beans or chickpeas—it will actually prevent other, higher-glycemic foods in the meal from causing inflammatory spikes in blood sugar and insulin levels. And, clinical studies show that RS even improves long-term insulin sensitivity, thanks to its probiotic, fermentation-increasing effects in the digestive system.

Like omega-3s, RS also possesses the rare ability to make you burn more body fat, as shown by the remarkable results of a small but well-designed clinical trial. The authors found that when participants enjoyed a meal containing a small amount of RS, the rate at which their bodies burned (oxidized) body fat increased by more than 20 percent—for an amazing 24 hours!

3. *Phytonutrient pigments:* The pigments that color beans—chiefly the same kinds of anthocyanins that color berries—are also potent antioxidant, anti-inflammatory agents. Anthocyanin phytonutrients—of which beans are surprisingly rich sources—are known to help control blood sugar modestly, and moderate the inflammatory impact of dietary sugars and standard starches.

4. *Starch blockers (amylase inhibitors):* Beans contain phytonutrients called amylase inhibitors, which block the action of the enzyme (amylase) needed to digest starches. Hypothetically, this effect should help prevent digestion of some of the starch in beans themselves, and of the starch in other foods eaten with beans.

However, I've listed amylase inhibitors last on the list of bean benefits, because it is not clear how effective the amylase inhibitors in whole beans—versus supplemental amylase inhibitors—are. Measurable weight loss resulting from dietary amylase inhibitors has been confirmed only in clinical trials testing supplements containing purified phaseamolin, an amylase inhibitor extracted from white kidney beans.

Among natural, unprocessed foods, beans contain the highest percentages of resistant starch, followed, at some distance, by whole, unrefined grains. The high levels of resistant starch in beans and whole grains could explain why, in population studies, people who get more of their protein from these complementary plant foods than from meats enjoy healthier body mass indices. No doubt their fiber also plays a significant role in preventing weight gain.

The healthiest members of the legume family—beans, lentils, and chickpeas—offer perfectly proportionate blends of resistant starch, fiber, protein, and antioxidant, anti-inflammatory phytonutrients. As a consequence, legumes exert as strong an effect on blood sugar regulation as any drug yet developed, without harmful side effects.

Legumes also offer a great, weight-controlling source of protein, although they can't replace the benefits of omega-3-rich fish. Legumes also come in a wide variety of flavors, shapes, sizes, and textures, lending themselves to a broad range of uses, and making it easy to choose one compatible with other elements of a meal.

Choose from popular varieties like black beans, white beans, pinto beans, kidney beans, red beans, chickpeas, and lentils to keep your diet both interesting and healthy.

The Least Glycemic Legume of All

An uncommon—but easily obtainable—legume from the Indian subcontinent may be the best bean of all, in terms of making the least impact on blood sugar. This legume is a lentil, known as chana gram dal, and hails from a distinct variety of the same plant that gives us plump yellow chickpeas (*Cicer arietinum*).

However, the chana dal variety of chickpea is much smaller and darker, and also higher in fiber and phytonutrients. Indian grocers call these two types of chickpea desi (chana dal) and kabuli (standard yellow chickpeas). While standard chickpeas rank relatively low on the glycemic index, chana dal ranks even lower, making it a superstar among the many blood-sugar-stabilizing stars in the legume family.

See our Resource Guide for Internet and direct mail sources of chana dal.

SUPERGROUP #8: LOW-FAT PROBIOTIC DAIRY FOODS WITH CALCIUM FOR WEIGHT LOSS AND BONE HEALTH

FUNCTIONAL WEIGHT CONTROL FACTOR: Nutriceutical Obesity-Fighters
TOP CHOICE: Low-Fat Yogurt
RUNNERS-UP: Low-Fat Kefir, Acidophilus Milk

Folks over 50 may remember when yogurt was an obscure item, found only in hippie communes and ethnic grocery stores. Then, along with many other important cultural innovations of the '60s era, yogurt began to move into the mainstream. By the mid-1970s, low-fat yogurt had begun to acquire popularity—especially among women—as a "diet food." Not because it was perceived to have any direct correlation to weight loss, but as a lower-calorie alternative to standard, higher-calorie lunch fare such as meat-and-cheese sandwiches or burgers and fries.

While the evidence is mixed, many studies indicate that both supplemental calcium and calcium-rich dairy foods promote weight loss. As the authors of one review of the scientific literature put it, "Each 300 mg increment in regular calcium intake is associated with approximately 1 kg [2.2 pounds] less body fat in children and 2.5–3.0 kg [5.5–6.6 pound] lower body weight in adults. Taken together these data suggest that increasing calcium intake by the equivalent of two dairy servings per day could reduce the risk of overweight substantially, perhaps by as much as 70 percent."

My confidence in the weight-loss powers of low-fat dairy foods is bolstered by important clues showing how calcium and other compounds in dairy foods would and should work to aid weight control.

Thanks to research conducted over the past decade, it appears likely that low-fat dairy foods possess the power to aid weight control, independent of their role as low-calorie substitutes for denser, higher calorie foods, which may be partly due to their calcium content.

According to a study conducted at the University of Tennessee, calcium exerts several beneficial effects:

◆ Calcium stored in fat cells plays an important role in fat storage and breakdown.

▼

◆ Higher calcium diets favor the burning of existing body fat over storage.

◆ High-calcium diets allow the body to keep burning food to create body heat (thermogenesis), even when calorie intake is relatively low. This is important to remember because when we are dieting and have cut our caloric intake, the body senses it and can go into a "starvation mode," in which it tenaciously clings to our body fat by slowing down our metabolism.

That said, when researchers compared the effects of diets containing comparable amounts of calcium, the results showed that dairy foods promoted weight loss more strongly than could be accounted for by their calcium content alone. As the authors of a 2004 review of the scientific literature said, "Notably, dairy sources of calcium markedly attenuate [reduce] weight and fat gain and accelerate fat loss to a greater degree than do supplemental sources of calcium."

Researchers attribute the greater weight-loss effect of dairy foods to two compounds in milk:

◆ Whey protein, which enhances glucose transport and inhibits production of angiotensin II, a bodily compound that promotes creation of body fat

◆ Branched-chain amino acids, which are known to help conserve muscle mass

Both of these nutriceutical factors interact synergistically with calcium to discourage deposition of calories as body fat. In other words, while adequate calcium consumption is critical to effective weight control, dairy foods seem to be the best calcium source for fighting the battle of the midriff bulge.

Top Choice: Low-Fat Yogurt

Making my top choice in the low-fat dairy category was easy. I say this only because the greatest number of studies has been done with yogurt. However, I also personally believe that kefir is as outstanding a healthy food as yogurt.

One of the clinical trials showing the greatest positive effect of dairy foods tested the effects of yogurt versus supplemental calcium. The results were very encouraging:

- Participant who ate yogurt lost about 10 pounds of fat, compared to only six pounds in the supplemental calcium group.

  ▼

- The waists of those who ate yogurt shrank by more than an inch and a half, compared with a loss of only about a quarter of an inch in waist size among the group taking calcium supplements. While the yogurt group did get more total calcium, they did much better than their higher intake—an extra 650 mg per day—would explain, especially in two months.

  ▼

- An impressive 60 percent of the yogurt eaters' weight loss was in the form of lost abdominal fat, whereas only 26 percent of the supplement group's loss was in the form of lost abdominal fat. Remember that abdominal fat is the hardest to lose, and that its fat cells pour out a constant stream of toxic, pro-inflammatory messenger chemicals (cytokines) that threaten overall health and greatly lessen the prospects for successful weight control.

  ▼

- Yogurt was about twice as effective at preserving muscle: the only kind of tissue that burns calories while your body is at rest.

Yogurt has many healthful properties, aside from its potential as a slimming food, thanks to both the "starter" cultures (*S. thermophilus* and/or *L. bulgaricus*) that turn milk into yogurt, and the "probiotic" bacteria often added to yogurt during production: *Bifidobacterium, L. acidophilus, L. rhamnosus,* and/or *L. reuteri.* (Unlike antibiotics, which poison disease bacteria, "probiotic" bacteria compete with disease bacteria in the gut and hamper their ability to cause mischief.) Both categories of beneficial bacteria promote good digestion, boost immune function, and increase resistance to infection. Regular consumption of probiotic-rich foods like yogurt seems to help lower cholesterol and prevent vaginal yeast infections, upper respiratory infections, ulcers, and certain cancers.

Whenever possible, choose organic yogurt, since conventional milk and dairy products often contain residues of growth hormones (used to increase cows' milk production) and antibiotics, which are given to cows to prevent the teat infections (mastitis) caused by the strain of supernormal milk production. Avoid yogurt that contains thickeners and stabilizers, which are fillers used to mask low-quality product, and choose unsweetened yogurt. Added sugars and fruits may impair survival of the cultures that make yogurt and other cultured dairy foods (kefir, acidophilus milk) so much more healthful than plain milk products. To make plain yogurt tastier, add your own fresh fruits and berries, sprinkle with nuts or seeds, and top off with a dash of cinnamon.

Runners-Up: Low-Fat Kefir and Acidophilus Milk

◆ **Kefir:** Along with a surfeit of death and destruction, the nomadic horsemen of Genghis Khan's world-beating Golden Horde also carried west primitive forms of both democracy and "probiotic" nutrition. Facing long days in the saddle with no time to forage for food, Mongol riders carried mare's milk in leather sacks, where it fermented to produce a thick, acidic beverage called koumiss. Thankfully, today's variation on the Mongol cavalry's durable equine drink– called kefir–is probably more healthful, and definitely far more appealing. (Kefir is pronounced keh-FEER, although "KEE-fur" is a very common pronunciation.) Descendants of the Mongol hordes, who settled in Russia's southern Caucasus Mountains, developed an heir to koumiss called "kefir," a thick, cultured milk beverage with a refreshing tang.

   Kefir is made by combining milk with a mixture of benign yeast and lactobacillus bacterial cultures called "kefir grains." The cultures release the small amount of carbon dioxide, alcohol, and aromatic compounds that give kefir its slightly fizzy, tangy taste.

   In addition to delivering live, beneficial probiotic cultures, commercial kefir often contains added inulin or fructoligosaccharides: types of long-chain carbohydrates upon which beneficial bacteria thrive. Kefir also contains special carbohydrates (polysaccharides) called kefiran, whose physiological effects explain some of its bountiful health benefits.

   Modern research indicates that kefir can stimulate the immune system, enhance lactose (milk sugar) digestion, and inhibit tumors, fungi, and pathogens, including the *Helicobacter pylori* bacteria that causes most ulcers. Accordingly, it is not uncommon for Russian and Central Asian physicians to prescribe kefir for a wide range of conditions, including high cholesterol, allergies, metabolic syndrome, tuberculosis, cancer, and gastrointestinal disorders.

Many natural food stores and most major supermarkets carry kefir, and I hope that it won't be long before the big conventional chains imitate their example. As with yogurt, avoid products with added sugars. Buy plain, unsweetened kefir and add berries or other high-fiber, low glycemic fruits for flavor. I like to flavor kefir with a splash of high-antioxidant açaí juice, pomegranate juice, or a shot of "green" drink made from wheat/barley grass or blended baby greens.

▼

◆ **Acidophilus milk:** As its name implies, acidophilus milk is simply milk to which a beneficial probiotic bacteria–*L. acidophilus*–has been added. However, unlike yogurt and kefir, acidophilus milk is not allowed to ferment and thicken. As a result, acidophilus milk doesn't taste much different than standard milk. If you are going to drink milk, or use it as an ingredient in recipes that do not involve much heat–too much of which would kill the beneficial bacteria–it makes sense to choose acidophilus milk.

SUPERGROUP #9: **OLD-FASHIONED WHOLE GRAINS**

FUNCTIONAL WEIGHT CONTROL FACTORS: Fiber, Anti-inflammatory
Antioxidants, and Other Phytonutrient Obesity-Fighters
TOP CHOICES: Buckwheat, Oats
RUNNER-UP: Barley

Readers of my prior books know that I am no fan of the high-glycemic carbohydrates—sugars and refined grain products—that dominate the standard American diet.
In fact, I hold them (along with a lack of omega-3 essential fatty acids) responsible for
the vast majority of health problems, including type 2 diabetes and obesity currently
plaguing much of the Western world. As we have learned, these foods raise blood
sugar quickly and sharply, provoking an insulin response that ultimately leads to carbohydrate cravings. So you may be wondering, given my concerns about carbohydrates, why would I include carbohydrate-rich grains in a list of recommended foods
for weight loss?

The answer lies in the critical distinction between high-glycemic, fiber-deficient
refined grain foods—such as the vast majority of bread, including so-called "whole
grain" bread, pasta, cookies, crackers, chips, and pastries—and low-glycemic, high-
fiber whole grains.

Several very large studies that examined links between the intake of whole grains
and weight control all came to the same conclusion: people who eat more whole
grain foods are less likely to be overweight.

For example, in 2003 and 2004, researchers at Harvard University published the
results of two studies examining eating patterns and alterations in weight. One analysis looked at more than 27,000 men over an eight-year period (1986–1994). The in-
vestigators reported finding that men who consumed more whole grains consistently
weighed less than men who consumed less whole grains.

A companion study analyzed the links between weight gain among 74,091 American nurses over a 10-year period (1984–1994), and it produced similar findings. The
women with the highest intake of high-fiber, whole-grain foods enjoyed the least
weight gain, while those with the highest intake of refined-grain foods experienced
the greatest risk of weight gain.

More important, the results of these large observational studies make sense in the context of the sound physiological reasons why high-fiber whole grains should aid weight control:

♦ High-fiber whole grains satisfy hunger far better, more quickly, and for a longer period of time than refined flour products.

▼

♦ Whole grains appear to increase insulin sensitivity, both in people with normal glucose tolerance and in those with impaired glucose tolerance.

▼

♦ The indigestible fibers in whole grains prevent blood sugar from rising quickly or to high levels in response to the digestible carbohydrates in grains.

▼

♦ Whole grains contain the same kinds of beneficial, anticancer lignan fibers—especially enterlactone—found in flaxseed. Enterlactone improves blood sugar control and retards the processes leading to insulin resistance (refined grain products contain little or none of this lignan).

▼

♦ In addition to fiber, the outer or bran layer of grains—which is found only in whole grain products—is rich in minerals, antioxidants, lignans, polyunsaturated fatty acids, stanols, and other beneficial phytonutrients.

▼

♦ Whole grains rival colorful fruits and vegetables as substantial sources of antioxidants, some of which promote burning of body fat and help moderate blood sugar levels.

Top Choice: Buckwheat

Buckwheat is incredibly nutritious and healthful, but ranks "low" on the glycemic index and "medium" on the glycemic load index. Like beans, much of the starch in buckwheat is fiberlike "resistant starch," which, along with buckwheat's unique proteins, helps reduce blood sugar levels both during and long after meals.

Buckwheat delivers more protein than rice, wheat, millet, or corn, and, unlike these grains, it contains lysine and arginine: two of the eight essential amino acids the body uses to make protein. And buckwheat contains no potentially problematic

Do You Have a Wheat Allergy?

Although the statistics are small, about one person in 133 has an allergy to gluten, a substance found in wheat and other grains (*oats* have traditionally been considered to be toxic to those with a wheat or gluten allergy, but recent scientific studies have shown otherwise.)

Interestingly, difficulty processing wheat gluten appears to primarily affect people of European (especially Northern European) descent, and more women than men appear to be affected, although it also appears that a wide variety of ethnic groups can also be affected. This allergy-like condition is insidious because it can produce a wide range of diverse symptoms—including many unrelated to digestion—and it can appear suddenly, at any stage of life.

If you have any family history of wheat or gluten allergy, it is wise to be tested. The extreme manifestation of this allergy is celiac disease, which can do silent damage to your intestines and cause malnutrition long before you experience symptoms. If you suspect that you may be gluten intolerant and need to learn more, log on to www.celiac.com for a comprehensive, in-depth discussion of this disease, including how to be correctly diagnosed.

Over the years I have observed that many of my patients may have a very low-grade wheat or gluten allergy. This is manifested as a slight increase in subclinical inflammation and complaints of fatigue. This is why I do not recommend wheat or other high-gluten grains in this book, as I believe a very large percentage of us are negatively affected at some level by these grains.

gluten—the biggest source of protein in wheat, rye, and barley—making it totally safe for people with problems digesting gluten.

In addition, buckwheat offers unique properties that make it a great antiglycemic weight-control ally and generally healthful in several ways:

- Buckwheat is by far the richest food source of rare carbohydrate compounds called fagopyritols—especially D-chiro-inositol—which, in diabetic rats, reduces blood sugar levels very substantially.

▼

- Buckwheat proteins make it one of the best cholesterol-lowering foods.

▼

- Buckwheat is low in total fat, and much of it (30–45 percent) is the monounsaturated type, the same type of fat that makes olives and olive oil so cardioprotective.

▼

- Buckwheat proteins partially inhibit angiotensin-converting enzyme (ACE), a protein that narrows the blood vessels, thereby reducing blood pressure.

▼

- Buckwheat contains more minerals—especially zinc, copper, and manganese—than cereal grains, and they are also more readily absorbed from buckwheat.

▼

- Like oats—and unlike most grains, whose fiber is largely the insoluble type—a considerable portion of buckwheat's fiber is soluble, which reduces blood cholesterol levels and the risk of colon cancer.

▼

- Buckwheat is rich in anti-inflammatory, antioxidant polyphenols, especially rutin, which reduces blood pressure and strengthens blood vessel walls, thereby helping to prevent hemorrhoids and varicose veins.

Although it is used as a grain, buckwheat is really the seed of a rhubarblike plant. Most of us know buckwheat as an ingredient in pancakes, or as "kasha"–the Eastern European name for roasted buckwheat groats, whose nutty flavor make kasha a delicious side dish. Many Eastern European cooks steam kasha in stock with onions, oil, and fresh parsley. I make hot cereal by cooking a blend of buckwheat and oats in water, and top the hearty result with berries, sesame seeds, or ground flaxseeds, and cinnamon for maximum nutritional and blood sugar stabilizing effects.

In Asia, buckwheat is usually enjoyed in the form of soba noodles, which are made with buckwheat flour, delicious alternatives to wheat pasta that take only about five minutes to cook. You can find soba noodles in Asian markets, natural food stores, and on the Internet. When I'm pressed for time, I can make a delicious accompaniment to my grilled salmon in 20 minutes by mixing basil pesto, pan-roasted pine nuts, sautéed onions, and steamed vegetables with hot soba noodles. Don't be afraid of the word "noodle." Soba noodles rank 46 on the glycemic index—and anything under 50 is considered to be a low-glycemic food.

Top Choice: Oats

Oats are most often identified as "the heart-healthy grain," but the same cholesterol-lowering beta-glucan fibers that make oats—and barley—good for cardiovascular health also offer considerable help in achieving weight control. And both of these whole grains provide excellent satiety, a great preventive benefit against overeating.

It turns out that in addition to its heart-healthy effects, the beta-glucan fiber in oats and also barley exerts beneficial antiglycemic effects as well. The results of a controlled clinical trial published in 2002 showed that diabetics given oatmeal, oat bran, or foods fortified with beta-glucan registered far lower and slower rises in blood sugar when compared with volunteers who consumed the same amount of white rice or bread. For individual servings I recommend one-half cup of cooked oats (in any form).

When choosing oats look for the following varieties:

1. Whole groats. These are oats that look like a large grain of rice. They are oats in their most natural unprocessed state. They may be cooked the same way as brown rice and make an excellent rice substitute for stir-fries, risottos, soups, chowders, and stews.

2. Steel-cut oats. Whole oat groats that have been cut into smaller pieces but otherwise unprocessed. Cook as you would whole oats. Can be used as a breakfast cereal or as a replacement for less desirable grains.

3. Old-fashioned oatmeal. These are whole oats that have been "rolled" or flattened. All nutrients are intact; the rolling enables them to cook more quickly. Oatmeal or rolled oats make an excellent breakfast cereal and are also a delicious addition to soups and chowders.

Runner-Up: Barley

Barley isn't nearly as popular as oats in American culinary culture, with the exception of hearty barley soups for cold days. Providing you have no problem with gluten, barley deserves a greater presence on our tables. Barley is both delicious and nutritious. It was a staple grain in ancient Greece, whose athletes relied heavily on barley-rich diets. And, ancient Rome's gladiators followed the Greeks' example so closely that they were called "barley eaters."

Hulled barley is the preferred type, since it retains its healthful, high-fiber bran (only the indigestible hull of the barley grain is removed). Pot, or "scotch" barley is more refined than the hulled barley, but it still retains more of the bran layer than the pearled type. Pearled barley is steamed and polished to remove almost all of the bran, and is not recommended.

Most important, barley is a low-glycemic grain that is high in both **soluble** and insoluble fiber.

◆ Soluble fiber is important because it lowers blood cholesterol levels.
▼

◆ Soluble fiber interacts with bile acids (compounds made by the liver from cholesterol) that are needed to correctly digest fat.
▼

◆ Soluble fiber slows down the rate of speed in which food leaves the stomach, thus exerting a stabilizing effect on blood glucose levels.
▼

◆ Insoluble fiber–commonly called "roughage"–promotes a healthy digestive tract and reduces the risk of cancers affecting it (e.g., colon cancer).
▼

◆ This high fiber content helps to speed food through the digestive track, helping to protect against cancer.
▼

◆ Barley is a good source of selenium, also shown to help reduce the risk of colon cancer.
▼

◆ Barley is cardioprotective thanks to its content of the B vitamin niacin.
▼

◆ It provides high concentrations of tocotrienols, the "super" form of vitamin E.
▼

◆ It contains antioxidant lignans; women who consume lignans (also present in high levels in flax and sesame seed) are less likely to develop breast cancer.

Oats' Artery-Protecting Antioxidants

Oats, oat bran, and oatmeal all contain beta-glucan: a special type of fiber with potent cholesterol-lowering powers. Lowering high cholesterol levels significantly reduces the risk of cardiovascular disease and stroke, and in people with cholesterol levels above 220 mg/dl, daily consumption of the amount of fiber in one bowl of oatmeal (three grams) can lower total cholesterol by up to 23 percent.

Now, thanks to recent research at Tufts University, we know that oats contain unique antioxidants called avenanthramides, phenol compounds like the potent antioxidants found in fruits and vegetables. Not only do oats' avenanthramides reduce the risk of cardiovascular disease by preventing free radicals from damaging LDL cholesterol, they also hinder the processes underlying the very first stage of atherosclerosis, in which immune (monocytes) cells stick to artery walls. In other words, there are many ways that eating oats can promote a healthy heart!

Barley adds hearty flavor and heft to soups, or you can cook it in stock with chopped onions and garlic and enjoy it as a side dish seasoned with your favorite herbs and spices. To reduce the cooking time, soak barley overnight. Barley also makes an excellent accompaniment to salmon and poultry. Simmer in chicken stock, add sautéed garlic and onion, a pinch of saffron, and a healthy sprig of fresh rosemary for a delightful risotto.

In moderation, buckwheat, oats, and barley can provide a good source of fiber and low-glycemic carbohydrates. But remember, when we discuss whole grains, we mean *whole* grains–not processed or adulterated in any way. And we don't mean "instant" anything: Instant and quick-cooking grains have had the benefits processed right out of them. Whole grains have a nutty flavor and a chewy texture. Unfortunately, most Westerners choose refined wheat flour as their grain of choice. This is a high-glycemic, low-fiber food and not recommended for the following reasons:

◆ The calorie content of refined white flour actually increases about 10 percent because of everything else that has been taken out.

◆ An average of 66 percent of the B vitamins has been removed.

- An average of 70 percent of all minerals has been removed.
- Seventy-nine percent of the fiber has been removed.
- An average of 19 percent of the protein has been removed.

Until recently, the amount and activity of antioxidants in whole grains has been grossly underestimated. However, a team of Cornell University researchers turned conventional wisdom on its head with a series of studies designed to tease out the actual, medically significant antioxidant capacity of whole and refined grains. They found that whole grains contain about as much or more antioxidant capacity as fruits and vegetables.

Researchers also found that more than 80 percent of a whole grain's antioxidant content is in the bran and germ, the layers that get removed when grains are refined.

The Cornell team's findings may explain why populations eating diets high in fiber-rich whole grains enjoy consistently lower risks of colon cancer, while clinical trials that have focused on fiber alone yield inconsistent results. It seems likely that the synergistic effects of all the nutrients in whole grains—including their antioxidants—account for the clear anticancer effects of whole grains.

SUPERGROUP #10: **VIBRANT VEGETABLES**

FUNCTIONAL WEIGHT-CONTROL FACTORS: Fiber, Low-calorie/Low-Glycemic Nutrition, Anti-inflammatory Antioxidants, and Other Phytonutrient Obesity-Fighters

TOP CHOICES: Garlic, Spinach, Kale, Broccoli Sprouts, Cruciferous Vegetables

RUNNERS-UP: Aromatic Culinary Herbs (e.g., Parsley, Mint, Rosemary, Thyme, Basil, Oregano)

Brightly colored vegetables are a special, slimming gift from Mother Nature's antioxidant/anti-inflammatory storehouse. Consequently, they deserve a place of distinction on your plate.

My top choices scored highest on the ORAC scale—a scientific measurement that allows us to see the antioxidant value of each vegetable and fruit. Colorful vegetables like spinach, broccoli, cabbage, and kale are very low in digestible carbohydrates, very high in fiber, and positively packed with antioxidants and other protective phytochemicals.

These vegetables are also very high in fiber, which as we know not only makes us feel full faster and longer, but also moderates the blood sugar impact of any sweet or starchy foods in a meal. This is important because according to a study conducted by the Department of Food Science and Nutrition, University of Minnesota, and published in the March 2005 issue of *Nutrition,* the average fiber intake of adults in the United States is less than half the recommended levels. And it is lower still among those who follow currently popular low-carbohydrate diets, such as Atkins and South Beach. This is critically important because the study further states what we all know—that there is strong epidemiologic support that dietary fiber intake prevents obesity. For healthy weight loss, we must have a form of low-glycemic fiber-rich carbohydrate at each meal and snack to accompany our quality protein and "good" fats.

Studies have found that individuals who regularly follow a dietary pattern low in total calories, saturated fat, and refined carbohydrates, moderate in whole grains, and high in vegetables and fruits reaped long-term health benefits and did not have struggles with weight control. The opposite was true for those individuals with a low intake of fruits and vegetables. These people all had a high BMI (body mass index). As we have mentioned, successful weight management is not just about what not to eat—it is equally important to eat the foods that are proven to help you lose weight and keep it off, such as plenty of fresh vegetables and fruit.

Top Choice: Garlic

Garlic is a superstar member of the allium family, which also contains onions, leeks, chives, shallots, and scallions. Garlic contains a special compound known as allicin, which must be crushed to be activated. Cooking pretty much destroys allicin, so use raw, crushed garlic for greatest health benefits. Garlic contains many different sulphur-rich compounds and provides many health benefits including

- the ability to lower total cholesterol while raising the HDL (good) cholesterol
- reduces toxins
- provides antifungal and antibacterial protection
- reduces the risk of certain cancers, particularly stomach-related
- reduces the risk of blood clots, the leading cause of stroke and heart attack
- lowers blood pressure
- lessens the risk of atherosclerosis (hardening of the arteries)
- has powerful anti-inflammatory activity

It is the last bullet point that is of greatest interest to those seeking to lose weight. However, if we are carrying extra weight, the additional benefits—especially the blood pressure, stroke, and cardiovascular protection—should be noted. As we know, being overweight places us at a significantly greater risk for these diseases.

Garlic and other members of the allium family contain compounds that inhibit the production of enzymes responsible for creating the inflammatory prostaglandins and thromboxanes (two types of autocrine hormones known as eicosanoids that produce inflammation in the body). Enjoy garlic daily, raw in salads and lightly sautéed in olive oil with any of the delightful vegetables listed here.

Top Choice: Spinach and Kale

Spinach and kale are deeply colored leafy vegetables containing the powerful carotenoids that are closely related to astaxanthin, the powerful antioxidant/anti-inflammatory that gives salmon its rich pink or red color. These dark leafy greens also contain other antioxidants such as lutein that work with the carotenoids to help protect our eyes from macular degeneration and cataracts, heart disease, and other age-related problems. Kale also contains sulforaphane and indoles that may help prevent cancer.

Top Choice: Broccoli Sprouts

Broccoli sprouts contain important anti-inflammatory phytonutrients–glucosinolates and isothiocyanates–and they are especially rich in glucoraphanin, a substance that boosts the body's antioxidant defense systems, as well as compounds that have been shown to reduce the risk of breast and colon cancer. Broccoli sprouts also act as an antibacterial agent against *Helicobacter pylori,* an organism associated with causing stomach ulcers. As reported in the May 10, 2004, edition of *Time,* a recent study indicates that eating broccoli sprouts may cut the risk of stroke, high blood pressure, and cardiovascular disease. If we are overweight our risk of these is elevated.

Top Choice: Cruciferous Vegetables

The cruciferous vegetables include broccoli, cauliflower, cabbage, Brussels sprouts, bok choy, and the aforementioned kale. This family of vegetables contains many components that have been linked to lower cancer risk, including glucosinolates, crambene, indole-3-carbinol and, especially, isothiocyanates (which are derived from glucosinolates–see broccoli sprouts, above). In fact, there is so much data about their disease-preventive effects, they are prominently featured on the American Institute for Cancer Research's website (www.aicr.org).

One of the important phytonutrients in this group, sulforaphane, has actually been found to be able to block the growth of breast cells that were already cancerous, and another, isothiocyanate, stimulates our bodies to break potential carcinogens down and prevent normal cells from becoming cancerous cells. In addition, the entire cruciferous family offers extremely powerful antioxidant and anti-inflammatory protection–making this entire group an ideal choice for the Perricone Weight-Loss Diet.

Runners-Up: Aromatic Culinary Herbs

Ounce for ounce, the culinary herbs win the antioxidant rating game hands down. The only reason they are not a top choice is because, as a rule, we consume them in much smaller quantities.

All herbs and spices provide exceptional antioxidant and anti-inflammatory protection. Use herbs and spices liberally by adding them to as many meals as possible. This will decrease inflammation and increase the flavor quotient.

As I said at the beginning of this chapter, my goal was to give you options. The foods in these 10 SuperGroups give you a huge variety of foods and unlimited combinations and menu choices. Unfortunately, that's not quite enough to keep your body at peak performance. In the next chapter, you'll find out what supplements you need to get you in top shape and keep you there.

Chapter 6

STEP TWO: 12 Nutritional Supplements That Facilitate Weight Loss While Maintaining Muscle Mass

Success is a science; if you have the conditions, you get the result.
— OSCAR WILDE

All of the SuperGroup foods in the last chapter were included because they help you lose weight and stay strong and healthy while you're getting thinner. The supplements included in this chapter are here for the same reasons.

The Perricone Weight-Loss Diet anti-inflammatory nutrients work in a special way to enhance loss of body fat, preserve muscle mass, and regulate levels of blood sugar and insulin, which are critical in the prevention and treatment of obesity.

These nutrients all have powerful anti-inflammatory and antioxidant activity. They're an important adjunct to any health regimen, and particularly important for a weight-loss program.

Many of my patients have asked me over the years if it is possible to get all of the necessary nutrients from a healthy diet. Unfortunately the answer is no. Alpha lipoic acid, for example, is one the most powerful and beneficial anti-inflammatory antioxidants and a very important nutrient for fighting aging and weight problems. However, there are no really adequate food sources for this nutrient. For optimum health and weight management we do need to supplement.

I always recommend that my patients take a complete spectrum of vitamins and minerals. In the 14-Day Perricone Weight-Loss Diet plan (Chapter 9), you will see that

I recommend you start the day with my Weight Management Program supplement, which contains all the major vitamins and minerals needed for optimum health as well as many of the special nutrients described below. You may also continue with your regular supplement program and add some or all of these nutrients as desired.

In this chapter I introduce my favorite "Superstar" supplements that are particularly relevant to weight loss. Fortunately, there are a number of outstanding supplements that really do help facilitate weight loss and maintain muscle mass. Each supplement has a distinct function, and they are all an important part of my own personal daily supplement regimen.

SUPERSTAR SUPPLEMENT #1: OMEGA-3 FISH OIL

Omega-3 fish oil supplements (as well as eating the fish itself) is extremely important to the success of any weight-loss plan, the Perricone Weight-Loss Diet included. In fact, it is difficult to overstate their many benefits, which has earned these essential fatty acids their own chapter in this book. I truly believe that they may be one of the most perfect anti-inflammatories we have discovered thus far. However, it is still important to take a variety of nutritional supplements to ensure optimum protection and benefit.

The incredible anti-inflammatory power of omega-3 essential fatty acids found in the high-fat fish and in fish oil can accomplish the following:

- reduce inflammation in all organ systems
- accelerate the loss of body fat
- elevate mood
- improve attention span
- stabilize blood sugar levels
- lower insulin levels
- create and maintain healthy serotonin levels
- stop the roller-coaster effects of the carbohydrate highs and lows
- decrease appetite
- increase radiance to skin
- increase health of immune system

- increase energy levels
- decrease symptoms and severity of rheumatoid arthritis
- reduce symptoms and severity of chronic skin conditions such as eczema
- decrease cardiovascular risk

Omega-3 Fish Oil Tips

- To avoid any dietary side effects from the omega-3 fish oils (such as belching or stomach upset), divide the dose into three. For example, if you are taking 3,000 mg per day of fish oil, take one 1,000 mg capsule with a meal three times per day.
- Even though fish oil is basically a "food," always check with your primary health-care professional before embarking on any new supplement. Any therapeutic intervention, even nutritional supplements, can be contraindicated in certain health conditions. This is especially true with heart patients. Numerous studies have shown that fish oil helps protect against sudden cardiac death and abnormal heart rhythms called arhythmias. However, according to a study in the June 2005 *Journal of the American Medical Association,* fish oil supplementation actually increased the rate of arhythmia among patients who had an implanted cardioverter defibrillator (ICD).

DOSAGE RECOMMENDATION: For a regular weight-loss diet, take one 1,000 mg capsule three times per day. If you need to lose a lot of weight or are trying to improve athletic performance, take three 1,000 mg capsules three times per day for a total of nine per day. Check with your physician before taking the larger dose.

SUPERSTAR SUPPLEMENT #2: ALPHA LIPOIC ACID (ALA)

Alpha lipoic acid is a potent antioxidant and anti-inflammatory. It is found naturally in the body, locked inside the mitochondria. Lipoic acid is part of an enzyme complex called the pyruvate dehydrogenase complex, making it intimately involved in the energy production of the cell. Alpha lipoic acid, like many of the other nutrients we will discuss in this chapter, including acetyl-L-carnitine, carnitine, and CoQ10, enhances our ability to metabolize food into energy.

Unlike many other antioxidants such as vitamin C, which is strictly water soluble, or vitamin E, which is strictly fat soluble, alpha lipoic acid is soluble in both water and fat. This means that alpha lipoic acid can go to all parts of the cell, including the lipid (fat) portions such as the cell plasma membrane, as well as the interior of the cell (known as the cytoplasm) where water-soluble chemicals reside. Because of this unique property, alpha lipoic acid is often referred to as "the universal antioxidant."

Needless to say, the amazing properties of alpha lipoic acid has placed it near and dear to my heart, both as a powerful ally in the antiaging realm and also as an integral part of the Perricone Weight-Loss Diet. On a cellular level alpha lipoic acid exerts a wide variety of positive actions, all of them anti-inflammatory. It also blocks the activation of transcription factor NfkB, as well, if not better than, any other antioxidant/anti-inflammatory thus far discovered.

In addition to its function as a powerful antioxidant/anti-inflammatory, alpha lipoic acid increases the body's ability to take glucose into the cells. This insulin-sensitizing effect is also seen in some of the other nutrients that we have discussed. These nutrients all work synergistically to increase sensitivity to insulin resulting in decreased blood sugar levels. Like carnitine and acetyl-L-carnitine, alpha lipoic acid is also very powerful in preventing glycation.

ALA works synergistically with CoQ10, carnitine, and acetyl-L-carnitine to protect and rejuvenate the mitochondria. If we recognize that an aging cell is characterized by *decreased* energy production, it is easy to see the importance of any substance that can increase energy levels in the cell, allowing the cells to repair themselves in the same way that young cells do. ALA also works synergistically with other antioxidants to raise levels of vitamins C and E, CoQ10, and glutathione in the cell.

Alpha Lipoic Tips

◆ In the metabolic cycle, alpha lipoic acid acts as a coenzyme in the production of energy by converting carbohydrates into energy (ATP).

◆ ALA is the only antioxidant that can boost cellular levels of glutathione, the body's most important antioxidant to overall health and longevity.

◆ Take with meals.

DOSAGE RECOMMENDATIONS: Because alpha lipoic acid is found only in trace amounts in food, it must be taken as a supplement. Twenty-five to 30 mg is adequate for a young healthy person. I recommend anywhere from 200 to 400 mg of alpha lipoic acid per day to my patients with specific health problems and to those who are trying to lose body fat.

SUPERSTAR SUPPLEMENT #3: ASTAXANTHIN

Astaxanthin comes from the microalgae *Haematococcus pluvialis,* found in abundance in arctic marine environments, and is a natural carotenoid (any of a class of yellow to red pigments, including the carotenes and the xanthophylls). Carotenoids are one of the most abundant molecules in the world and give nature its wide variety of colors—from carrots to flamingos. Astaxanthin is an amazingly powerful antioxidant and is often referred to as "red gold from the sea."

Astaxanthin is one of the xanthophyll group of the carotenoid family. Xanthophylls help to protect vitamin A and vitamin E and other carotenoids from oxidation. It is the most potent of all of the carotenoids—in fact, it is 10 times stronger than beta-carotene and 100 times stronger than vitamin E. Wild Alaskan salmon, lobster, rainbow trout, shrimp, crawfish, crab, and red caviar all owe their rich colors to their astaxanthin-rich diets—just one of the reasons wild salmon tops my SuperFood list. The variety of wild Alaskan salmon known as "sockeye" delivers the greatest amount of astaxanthin, with 4.5 mg per four-ounce serving. To put this in antioxidant perspective, 4.5 mg of astaxanthin is equal to 450 mg of vitamin E. Astaxanthin is also superior to many other antioxidants due to the unique role it may play in protecting the cell membrane.

Astaxanthin Tips

- Because astaxanthin has been proven to cross the blood–brain barrier (see carnitine), it offers protection to the brain, the central nervous system, and the eyes.
- It increases physical endurance and reduces muscle damage.
- It reduces eye fatigue and improves visual acuity.
- It provides wrinkle reduction by internal supplementation.

- It reduces hyperpigmentation (better known as age spots).
- It provides cytokine regulation; inhibiting the expression of inflammatory cytokines and chemokines.
- It improves gastric health and reduces infection/inflammation of *H. pylori,* spiral-shaped bacteria that can damage stomach and duodenal tissue, causing ulcers.

Astaxanthin is an exceptional anti-inflammatory, making it an important component of the Perricone Weight-Loss Diet. Its ability to protect muscles and increase physical endurance is a wonderful asset for everyone needing to start and maintain a regular exercise program. I strongly recommend supplementation–look for the AstaReal™ trademark on your bottle of astaxanthin supplements for potency and purity.

DOSAGE RECOMMENDATION: One to two capsules, 2 mg each, per day.

SUPERSTAR SUPPLEMENT #4: **CARNITINE**

Carnitine is a nutrient that was once classified as an amino acid, but we now know that is incorrect. Carnitine is a water-soluble nutrient, very much like a B vitamin, that allows us to convert fat into energy. Carnitine and its derivative, acetyl-L-carnitine (which we will discuss later), are two of the most important nutrients for weight loss. However, for carnitine to have optimum effect, we must have adequate essential fatty acids (such as omega-3s) present in the diet. Carnitine is critical for energy formation and an active metabolism. Small amounts of carnitine can be obtained from foods such as meats and dairy products, but to get an adequate supply we must take carnitine supplements.

You'll remember that fats provide an important source of energy within the body, especially for muscles such as the heart, as well as vital organs such as the liver. In order for fat to be turned into fuel, it has to be carried into the energy-producing portion of the cell known as the mitochondria. It is the role of carnitine to transport the fatty acids from our blood into the cell for this energy production.

Carnitine also provides antiaging benefits in that it enhances energy production in the cell, which is needed for cellular repair. Studies have also shown that carnitine helps prevent muscle loss during illness and also prevents the muscle loss associated with aging, known as sarcopenia. Carnitine is protective of liver function and enhances and protects the immune system, especially under stressful conditions.

Carnitine Tips

◆ For carnitine to have optimum effect, make sure you have an adequate omega-3 intake.

◆ Do not take carnitine in the evening as it may interfere with sleep.

◆ Carnitine may be taken with or without food.

◆ For better utilization of fat for energy take omega-3 fish oil with carnitine.

DOSAGE RECOMMENDATION: The recommended dose for an adult under the age of 30 without ill health or obesity is approximately 500 mg per day. For those who are obese or have other health problems, the recommendation is 1,500 to 2,000 mg per day, taken in 500 mg doses three or four times per day.

SUPERSTAR SUPPLEMENT #5: ACETYL-L-CARNITINE

Acetyl-L-carnitine is synthesized from carnitine by the addition of an acetyl group to the carnitine molecule. While this synthesis means that it cannot be found in food, the good news is that this form of carnitine can pass through the blood–brain barrier, which separates the blood vessels from the central nervous system. The barrier has a protective effect, but it can stop the passage of therapeutic substances along with the harmful ones. Since acetyl-L-carnitine can penetrate this barrier, it has a particularly beneficial effect on the brain cells. In fact, acetyl-L-carnitine is extremely neuroprotective and should be used on a daily basis to prevent the neurological decline seen with aging.

Like carnitine, acetyl-L-carnitine improves mitochondrial function, but to an even greater degree, because it can pass through the mitochondrial membrane. And like carnitine, acetyl-L-carnitine functions best when there is adequate dietary intake of omega-3 essential fatty acids. Acetyl-L-carnitine is a natural anti-inflammatory that enhances the effects of antioxidant systems within the body. These anti-inflammatory properties protect the cell plasma membrane (the cell's first line of defense) and prevent the conversion of arachidonic acid into inflammatory chemicals.

Acetyl-L-carnitine can also help repair the mitochondria, boost levels of the antioxidants glutathione and Coenzyme Q10, and work synergistically with alpha lipoic acid, another powerful antioxidant/anti-inflammatory. Both acetyl-L-carnitine and carnitine have been known to actually improve the lipid profile within our blood by reducing the level of triglycerides and raising levels of HDL (good) cholesterol.

Both forms of carnitine are important in a weight-loss regimen because they act as natural anti-inflammatories, and they aid in transportation of fats into the mitochondria to be burned. They also enhance the sensitivity of insulin receptors, helping to decrease blood sugar and circulating levels of insulin. As we have learned, high levels of insulin are inflammatory and "lock" our body fat in place.

Both carnitine and acetyl-L-carnitine help prevent glycation (see box on the next page).

Acetyl-L-Carnitine Tips

◆ Carnitine and acetyl-L-carnitine are *not* to be used by people with bipolar disease (manic depression) or those who are susceptible to seizures (epilepsy) unless recommended by their physician.

▼

◆ Do not take acetyl-L-carnitine after 3:00 P.M. to prevent any difficulties with sleeping.

▼

◆ Exercise naturally increases our levels of acetyl-L-carnitine; however, if we are obese, over 30, or have other health problems, it will not raise them to therapeutic levels; therefore supplementation is necessary.

▼

◆ Acetyl-L-carnitine may be taken with or without food.

▼

♦ For better utilization of fat for energy take omega-3 fish oil with carnitine.

DOSAGE RECOMMENDATION: 500 mg per day; however, individuals on a weight-loss program may take up to 1,500 mg daily.

The Damaging Effects of Glycation

Throughout this book, you have been advised to avoid high-glycemic foods as a surefire way to decrease inflammation and facilitate weight loss. However, there is another reason to steer clear of these foods. I have explained that these foods cause sudden spikes in blood sugar levels, resulting in the release of insulin into the bloodstream that then cause us to store, rather than burn, fat.

However, that is not the only negative byproduct. As we know, when sugars and starches are eaten, they cause a burst of inflammation throughout the body. These sugars (and foods that rapidly convert to sugar) can permanently attach to the collagen present in our skin and other parts of the body through a process known as "glycation". At the point of attachment, there is a small mechanism creating inflammation, which then becomes a source of inflammation in its own right. This inflammation produces enzymes that break down collagen, resulting in wrinkles. In addition to inflammation, glycation also causes cross-linking in our collagen, making it stiff and inflexible where it was once soft and supple.

But it is not just the skin we have to worry about. These "sugar-bonds" can occur throughout the body as we age. The sugar molecule attaches itself to our collagen as well as our arteries, veins, bones, ligaments, even our brains, resulting in the breakdown of organ systems and the deterioration of the body. Glycation creates "free radical" factories known as advanced glycation end products (AGEs), which also increase cellular inflammation. Because the Perricone Weight-Loss Diet is *anti-inflammatory*, it will prevent glycation, stop inflammation, keep the brain functioning properly, and facilitate weight loss. The alternative? Being wrinkled, depressed, and overweight.

SUPERSTAR SUPPLEMENT #6: CONJUGATED LINOLEIC ACID (CLA)

CLA is a fatty acid that is found in many of the foods we eat. At one time, beef and lamb were exceptional sources; however, when their diet was changed from grass to grain, levels of CLA dramatically decreased in meat and dairy products. When CLA is present, it is found in the fatty portion of milk. Drinking skim milk prevents us from receiving the benefits of CLA. However, since CLA levels are now so low in animal products, skim vs. full-fat milk is a moot point.

Conjugated linoleic acid, like many of the other nutrients in this chapter, has powerful antioxidant/anti-inflammatory activity. In fact, CLA has been rated as three times more powerful an antioxidant than vitamin E.

CLA is also a powerful aid in prevention and treatment of obesity. When taken in effective doses, CLA decreases body fat, especially in the area of the abdomen. There are several mechanisms of CLA's activity that accomplish these feats:

◆ CLA actually concentrates in the cell membrane, stabilizing it and thus preventing the breakdown of arachidonic acid into a pro-inflammatory prostaglandin. It helps the insulin receptors remain intact, thus increasing insulin sensitivity, which will then decrease blood sugar and circulating insulin levels.

▼

◆ Remarkably, studies show that CLA also helps block the absorption of fat and sugar into fat cells (adipocytes). It even induces a reduction in the actual size of the fat cells (one reason people gain weight as they age is that their fat cells literally become fatter).

▼

◆ A relatively recent and large-scale study published in the *Journal of Nutrition* showed that taking 3.4 grams of CLA a day for two years led to a small but significant decrease in body fat in overweight people. Interestingly, CLA appears to have no effect on the body fat of people who are not overweight.

In addition to the antioxidant, anti-inflammatory, and insulin-sensitizing actions of CLA, many studies show that CLA helps prevent muscle loss and weakness associated with aging and disease. This is one of the reasons CLA has long been a favorite supplement of athletes and body builders. What could be more exciting or encouraging than a supplement that shrinks body fat while increasing and preserving lean muscle mass?

CLA Tips

- When taken with sesame seeds, the effects of CLA are enhanced.
- The average diet provides no more than a gram (1,000 mg) of CLA per day.
- CLA may be taken with meals.

DOSAGE RECOMMENDATION: 1,000 mg, up to a maximum of 4,000 mg per day, taken in one or two doses.

SUPERSTAR SUPPLEMENT #7: COENZYME Q10 (CoQ10)

Coenzyme Q10, also called ubiquinone, is a powerful antioxidant/anti-inflammatory with many benefits for treating and preventing obesity. It acts similarly to acetyl-L-carnitine in that it assists in energy production within the mitochondria. As we have learned, energy production declines as a cell ages, and that means that the cell's ability to repair itself also declines. Working synergistically with acetyl-L-carnitine, carnitine, and alpha lipoic acid in the mitochondria, CoQ10 enhances the metabolism, giving us greater energy and endurance, and a greater ability to lose body fat, while preventing the energy decline seen in aging cells. CoQ10 also works synergistically with other antioxidants to elevate cellular levels of vitamins C and E and glutathione and to help regulate blood sugar and enhance insulin sensitivity. CoQ10 also maximizes the burning of foods for fuel, helping to normalize fats in our blood.

Hundreds of studies document the effectiveness of CoQ10 in protecting all vital organs of the body including the brain, heart, and kidneys. Because of its powerful anti-inflammatory effects, CoQ10 is extremely protective of the cardiovascular system. It keeps the heart muscle healthy and also prevents inflammation in the arteries, which leads to arteriosclerosis.

Although CoQ10 can be found in small amounts in fish such as sardines or salmon, as well as in nuts, I recommend supplementation for optimal antiaging and weight-loss benefits. CoQ10 supplementation is of particular importance for women because they tend to have lower levels than their male counterparts.

CoQ10 Tips

◆ This supplement should be taken by anyone over 40, as tissue levels of CoQ10 decrease as people get older.

◆ CoQ10 is best taken with food.

DOSAGE RECOMMENDATION: I recommend a minimum of 30 mg per day. For those with health problems, under the supervision and recommendation of their physician, up to 300 mg per day. About three weeks of daily dosing are necessary to reach maximal serum concentrations of CoQ10.

SUPERSTAR SUPPLEMENT #8: CHROMIUM

Chromium is a critical nutrient in our effort to control and reduce excess body fat. By supplementing our diets with chromium, we can effectively lower blood sugar and insulin levels–the key to the anti-inflammatory weight-loss diet. The reason people are overweight is because they're in an inflammatory state that has put a "lock" on their fat-burning mechanism. Our goal is to reverse this. Chromium helps decrease inflammation, thereby unlocking the enzymes that aid in fat metabolization. Chromium not only affects blood sugar and insulin levels, it can also help normalize blood lipids such as triglycerides and cholesterol, increasing levels of the HDL "good" cholesterol and lowering total cholesterol and triglycerides, making it cardioprotective.

Experts in the field of nutrition report that the general population of the United States is deficient in chromium, and low levels of chromium are associated with type 2 diabetes and cardiovascular disease. Studies have also been published noting that increased consumption of sugar depletes our body stores of chromium, placing us at further risk for hyperglycemia and hyperinsulinaemia (too much blood sugar, too much insulin).

Chromium Tips

◆ Chromium is an essential nutrient required for normal sugar and fat metabolism.

▼

◆ Chromium is important for energy production, and also plays a key role in regulating appetite, reducing sugar cravings, and lowering body fat.

▼

◆ Chromium absorption is made more difficult when milk, as well as foods high in phosphorus, are eaten at the same time.

▼

◆ Don't take chromium with foods rich in phytic acid (unleavened bread, raw beans, seeds, nuts, grains, and soy isolates) as this may decrease its absorption.

▼

◆ The recommended type of this supplement is chromium polynicotinate.

DOSAGE RECOMMENDATION: I suggest 100 micrograms (mcg) per day for the average person over 40 and up to 200 mcg per day for those on the Perricone Weight-Loss Diet.

Brewer's Yeast, a Natural Source of Chromium

Some experts believe that close to 90 percent of Americans do not get enough chromium in their diet. It is certainly possible that a widespread deficiency in chromium is contributing to the epidemic of metabolic disorder, obesity, and type 2 diabetes.

In addition to taking chromium supplements, we can also add brewer's yeast to our diet (don't confuse brewer's yeast with baker's yeast—they are entirely different substances). Brewer's yeast is actually used by brewers as the active yeast used to make beer. However, it can also be grown to make

nutritional supplements. In addition to helping the body to maintain normal blood sugar levels, brewer's yeast is also an excellent source of protein and the B-complex vitamins, which are critical to the health of our nervous and digestive systems for wound healing, to fight stress, chronic fatigue and depression, and for the health of our skin and liver.

Unfortunately, brewer's yeast has a rather unpleasant, bitter taste. Mixing it in a yogurt and berry smoothie might help to disguise the taste.

SUPERSTAR SUPPLEMENT #9: GAMMA LINOLENIC ACID (GLA)

GLA is an important omega-6 essential fatty acid. We have read throughout this book that the average Western diet has an excess of the omega-6 EFAs. And this is true when we are speaking of linolenic acid, found in many vegetable oils, grains, and seeds. However, GLA is an omega-6 that is well worth taking in a supplemental form. The body rapidly converts GLA into dihomogamma-linolenic acid (DGLA), the precursor of prostaglandin E1, a powerful anti-inflammatory hormone-like compound that helps to regulate inflammation, blood pressure, and many other bodily processes. Because of the increased production of prostaglandin E1, GLA has been found in many studies to lower total cholesterol, as well as lowering blood pressure. GLA can also increase the metabolic rate, an effect that causes the body to burn fat, resulting in weight loss.

The average American diet causes a deficiency of GLA because of the large amounts of trans fatty acids, sugar, red meats, and dairy products that are consumed. GLA is very difficult to find in the diet, but is found in high amounts in borage, black currant, and evening primrose oils.

GLA Tips

♦ Take GLA with meals to increase absorption.

▼

♦ GLA improves cell sensitivity to insulin, reducing our chance of developing diabetes, heart disease, and excess body fat.

▼

♦ Borage oil is the richest supplemental source of GLA.

▼

♦ As with omega-3 fish oil supplementation, results do not happen overnight and may take up to six months. Don't let this dissuade you from adding this vital essential fatty acid to your diet as soon as possible.

DOSAGE RECOMMENDATION: 200 to 400 mg of GLA per day—one to two 1,000 mg of borage oil.

SUPERSTAR SUPPLEMENT #10: **GLUTAMINE**

Glutamine is an extremely important dietary supplement for anyone wishing to lose weight. It is an amino acid that is classified as "conditionally essential," meaning that we are able to synthesize it, but only within certain limits that are controlled by a variety of factors (including the dietary supply of the appropriate precursors and the maturity and health of the individual). Glutamine is primarily stored within muscles and is the body's most abundant amino acid. (Amino acids are the basic building blocks of a protein. There are 20 different amino acids commonly found in proteins. There are 8 essential amino acids: isoleucine, leucine, lysine, methionine, phenylalanine, threonine, tryptophan, and valine. Our bodies actually need 20 different amino acids, but we are able to make the other 12 kinds from these 8, which we must get from food.)

While the majority of the glutamine we need is synthesized in our muscle cells, we can also obtain a significant amount of glutamine from several dietary sources, including poultry, fish, dairy products, and legumes.

However, under certain stressful conditions, glutamine is used up very quickly and our body cannot make as much as it needs. For example, prolonged and intense cardiovascular workouts, such as running and aerobics, can cause the body to burn muscle for energy, exhausting our glutamine supply.

It appears that glutamine plays an important role in keeping the muscles functioning properly and in helping to reduce muscle deterioration. One reason is that glutamine is the only amino acid that contains two nitrogen molecules. Because of this additional molecule, glutamine can transport, or shuttle, the nitrogen to where it is needed most. Nitrogen is one of the building blocks of muscle cells; glutamine is the delivery system for getting the nitrogen to those cells. Glutamine can also transport excess nitrogen out of the body—a critical function because nitrogen can act as a toxin. The optimal state for muscle growth is when glutamine is working properly, and nitrogen intake is greater than nitrogen output.

When we are overweight and in an inflammatory state, we need even more glutamine—so the body breaks down the muscle tissue to get the extra glutamine it needs—and we lose muscle mass. Making sure we have enough glutamine enables us to both lose weight and retain muscle mass.

Glutamine plays a number of vitally important roles in many other functions as

Anabolic vs. Catabolic

The term "anabolic" means to build up tissue; the term "catabolic" means to break down tissue. Our goal is to always be in an anabolic state. Anabolic-stimulating substances are made by the body and they include the growth hormones and the sex hormones such as testosterone.

The catabolic state is also termed as "the clinical wasting syndrome or cachexia," a syndrome that is characterized by unintended and progressive weight loss, weakness, and low body fat and muscle. This catabolic state can occur in diseases such as cancer and AIDS.

Inflammation puts our body in a catabolic state even though we may not be seriously ill. The anti-inflammatory diet and anti-inflammatory supplements, such as alpha lipoic acid, CoQ10, and glutamine are extremely important forms of protection as we embark on a weight-loss program.

well. It is absolutely essential to the support of our immune system and immune response, where it is utilized by white blood cells. Glutamine is also anti-catabolic, which means that it is critical in the prevention of muscle breakdown caused by extreme stress, including physical trauma or injury, severe burns, disease, mental or psychic stress, overwork or overexertion, poor nutrition, and dieting.

Glutamine has such extraordinary anticatabolic properties that is has been used to help prevent stress ulcers in severe burns. Scientists have also found that patients who have had major surgery or trauma do not lose muscle mass during the recuperative period when they are given supplemental glutamine, even if they are inactive! This prevention of muscle breakdown is the reason that I so strongly recommend that you take glutamine throughout the day as part of the anti-inflammatory diet.

Glutamine is also very supportive of our digestive system. The health of the gut is of critical importance because it is the point of fuel and nutrient entry. Glutamine nourishes the cells that line the stomach, intestines, and digestive track, which actually use glutamine as a fuel. Studies have shown that supplemental glutamine may protect against aspirin-induced gastric lesions and enhance healing of painful peptic ulcers. In fact, an old folk remedy for ulcers is fresh cabbage juice—which is high in glutamine. Glutamine may also be helpful in healing the stomach problems arising from colitis and Crohn's disease. In summary, glutamine can be used whenever there are any stomach problems, as simple as overindulging in alcohol (alcoholic-induced gastritis) to ulcers, viral-induced diarrhea, or even severe problems such as inflammatory bowel disease.

It is difficult to overstate the importance of glutamine to our body's antioxidant system. In combination with other amino acids, *N-acetyl cysteine and glycine,* glutamine promotes the synthesis of *glutathione* in the liver. Glutathione is the body's primary antioxidant defense system; it is required for the smooth functioning of all cells. It is involved in protein synthesis, amino acid transport, and in the recycling of other antioxidants, such as vitamin C. In fact, it is so effective in preventing inflammation in the body that glutathione is being used to treat people with HIV infection who suffer from high levels of inflammation and body wasting.

Glutamine will reduce cravings for high-glycemic carbohydrates and will make your weight-loss program much easier. Glutamine can help prevent both depression and fatigue and can also help us synthesize neurotransmitters in the brain, which naturally relax us while elevating our mood. In the brain it is converted to glutamic acid and increases the concentration of GABA (gamma-aminobutyric acid). Both glutamic acid and GABA can be considered "brain fuel," as they are essential for normal mental function. Studies have also shown that glutamine supplementation helps prevent the damaging effects of alcohol on the brain and may also reduce alcoholic (as well as food) cravings.

Glutamine Tips

◆ Once mixed in water, glutamine deteriorates rapidly, so take it immediately upon mixing in the water.

▼

◆ Do not store glutamine solution, as it may become inactive or possibly toxic.

▼

◆ Mix fresh for each serving.

▼

◆ Check with your primary care physician before beginning any supplementation program—this is mandatory if you are being treated for any disease or kidney, liver, or other health problem, are pregnant, or nursing.

▼

- Glutamine may cause constipation in some individuals; to protect from this, increase your water and soluble fiber intake. This can be accomplished by adding one gram of pectin to a glass of water.

DOSAGE RECOMMENDATION: One-half teaspoon of glutamine dissolved in water three times a day.

SUPERSTAR SUPPLEMENT #11: MAITAKE MAGIC

The Maitake SX Fraction™ is a special supplement derived from the maitake mushroom. There is a solid body of scientific evidence establishing it as a powerful tool in preventing metabolic syndrome, a dangerous quartet of metabolic imbalances that increase our risk of cardiovascular disease and diabetes: 1) high blood pressure, 2) elevated levels of insulin, 3) excess weight (especially around the abdomen), and 4) "dyslipidemia" (low levels of HDL "good" cholesterol, high levels of LDL "bad" cholesterol, and high levels of triglycerides [metabolized dietary fats that end up in our blood, organs, and tissues]. Metabolic syndrome is a by-product of Americans' sedentary lifestyles in conjunction with an inflammatory diet high in sugars, starches, and processed "junk" foods.

The Maitake Grifron **SX-Fraction™** has been developed based on a newly discovered active fraction from the Maitake mushroom (*Grifola frondosa*) in collaboration with Harry G. Preuss, M.D., of Georgetown University. Dr. Preuss is also the highly regarded author of the book *Maitake Magic* (see Resource Guide).

The study at Georgetown University started in 1997 based on a previously discovered compound, X-Fraction, which Japanese scientists demonstrated had antidiabetic activity. Searching for a better compound, researchers developed an improved method to successfully fractionate and identify another active compound from maitake, named **SX-Fraction.™** Studies on **SX-Fraction™** have been conducted at Georgetown University and New York Medical College. Results show that **SX-Fraction™** does indeed possess a more potent ability to enhance insulin sensitivity for controlling blood sugar levels and lowering high blood pressure than X-fraction. This is another exciting, therapeutic tool to add to our arsenal of substances that can positively affect out-of-control blood sugar and all of its negative ramifications.

Leading experts believe that the Maitake **SX-Fraction**™ may be very helpful not only in prevention, but also for those who suffer from chronic disorders associated with the aging process due to malfunction of blood glucose/insulin metabolism.

A recent study conducted at four clinics in Japan gave 33 diabetic people, who were on a stable drug regimen, nine tablets of **SX-Fraction**™ daily. Both blood sugar and cholesterol markers were improved significantly. In addition, they lost six pounds in a two-month period, without dieting. While this is not dramatic, it is statistically significant and future studies may show that in addition to preventing metabolic syndrome, **SX-Fraction**™ may serve as a safe and reliable weight-loss supplement—even without additional behavior modifications, such as decreased caloric intake and increased exercise.

It appears that the Maitake **SX-Fraction**™ may be the first dietary supplement of this kind specifically targeting metabolic syndrome with abundant scientific validation behind it. And the research continues to this day.

Maitake SX-Fraction™ Tips

◆ Recent studies suggest that this active constituent may help maintain healthy cardiovascular function and a healthy circulatory system.

◆ For optimum effect take between meals.

DOSAGE RECOMMENDATION: I recommend that you select the Grifron SX-Fraction™ **of Maitake Mushroom Extract Supplement because this is the standardized product used in the studies. For general support for healthy blood sugar maintenance, take one tablet within 30 minutes after each meal. For maximum impact, you may double or triple the general dose.**

Polysaccharide Blend for Weight Loss

In addition to Maitake SX-Fraction™, there is also another substance with somewhat similar properties. Scientists at universities in the United States and Asia recently discovered a previously unknown class of polysaccharides (chains of linked sugar molecules) called alpha-glucans, which produce dramatic positive effects on the efficiency and integrity of the mitochondria.

Working with some of these researchers, I have formulated these polysaccharides into a nutritional food product known as polysaccharide peptide blend, or "PEP." One of its benefits is keeping the mitochondrial portion of the cell (where the food we eat is converted to energy in our bodies) healthy and functioning properly.

PEP food also contains the all-important essential fatty acids. One serving once a day delivers four groups of nutrients:

◆ *Lignans from flaxseed hulls:* These healthful, phyto-estrogenic fibers help to control blood sugar and insulin. They also help improve gastrointestinal health, thus enhancing absorption and elimination of foods, and they appear to enhance the antioxidant power and energy-generating capacity of the cells' mitochondria.

◆ *Amino acids and polypeptides:* The PEP blend contains all eight essential amino acids needed for making the proteins in our connective tissues, as well as 10 additional amino acids that exert beneficial effects on the energy-producing capacity of our cells.

◆ *Vitamins and minerals:* Selected essential nutrients with particular benefits on the body's antioxidant and tissue repair systems.

◆ *Dietary fibers:* Selected soluble and insoluble fibers to help control blood sugar and enhance digestion.

Like Maitake SX-Fraction, the effects of the PEP polysaccharide blend are physiologic, which means that unlike a drug, it works with the body to help maintain cellular integrity. I recommend that you include at least one of these polysaccharide formulas in your daily supplement routine. Some of the unique benefits include

◆ reduced inflammation throughout the body
◆ increases in the cells' uptake of glucose, thus reducing hyperinsulinemia (too much insulin) and metabolic syndrome
◆ increased physical and mental energy
◆ increased circulation in the muscles, heart, brain, and other organs
◆ vibrant, soft, supple skin
◆ increased production of fibroblasts, the cells that build tissues in the skin and elsewhere

SUPERSTAR SUPPLEMENT #12: **DIMETHYLAMINOETHANOL (DMAE)**

DMAE is a naturally occurring nutritional substance with powerful anti-inflammatory properties. It is found in fish, including wild Alaskan salmon, anchovies, and sardines. Back in the 1950s, DMAE was a prescription drug used as a treatment for central nervous system problems such as attention deficit disorder. Although it is no longer used for this purpose, it is being sold as a nutritional supplement for improving cognitive function, with additional benefits of improved memory and increased problem-solving ability. DMAE is important in the production of neurotransmitters, especially acetylcholine, which is essential in the communication from one nerve to another and between nerves and muscles. In order for your muscles to contract, the message must be sent from your nerves to your muscles via acetylcholine. DMAE also has membrane-stabilizing effects and can also help reduce body fat, most likely from its activity as a precursor to acetylcholine as well as its anti-inflammatory activity.

Taking DMAE as a supplement will not only improve your cognitive function, it will help increase skin firmness and muscle tone. In fact, recent studies have confirmed that topically applied DMAE lotion turned out to be extremely efficacious—in other words, it had positive effects on the skin, greatly increasing the appearance of radiance, tone, and firmness, while decreasing the micro-inflammation in the skin.

DMAE Tips

- For optimum health, beauty, and weight-loss benefits, I recommend eating fish rich in DMAE, taking DMAE supplements, as well as applying a topical lotion containing DMAE to face, neck, and body.

  ▼

- It is thought that DMAE can make epilepsy and bipolar depression worse; thus, it is advised that those with these health problems avoid DMAE.

  ▼

- DMAE can also be overstimulating for some people, perhaps causing muscle tension or insomnia, so individuals experiencing such difficulties are advised to discontinue use of DMAE.

  ▼

- Take with meals for optimum effect.

DOSAGE RECOMMENDATION: My recommended dose is 50 to 100 mg per day. For certain therapeutic uses, such as lowering cholesterol, larger doses may be recommended. As always, consult your physician.

The next chapter is the third step in the Perricone Weight-Loss Diet—The Anti-inflammatory Lifestyle. It's about how you live your life, how you treat yourself, and what you can do to keep your body and brain inflammation-free for optimum health, weight management, and well-being.

Chapter 7

STEP THREE: The Anti-inflammatory Lifestyle

Motivation is what gets you started. Habit is what keeps you going.
— JIM RYUN, THREE-TIME U.S. OLYMPIAN

ood isn't the only thing that makes us fat. An amazingly large number of factors from how much sleep we get to how much water we drink can trigger or inhibit the inflammatory response. This chapter will give you an overview of what you need to keep in mind to achieve optimum fat loss, but the bottom line is simple: treat yourself well and the weight will come off.

The Perricone Weight-Loss Diet is not just about the foods we do or do not eat. It is also about understanding the actions we do in our daily lives that are pro-inflammatory, and learning how to change them. Many have a direct link to obesity and weight gain, as well as accelerated aging, wrinkles, the thinning of skin, the killing of brain cells and shrinking of the brain, and a weakened immune system. In this chapter we are not only going to look at proven methods to reduce inflammation in the body and lose weight, we are also going to learn that these same strategies increase our sense of well-being.

ANTI-INFLAMMATORY BENEFITS OF EXERCISE

Let's start with physical activity. Exercise will not only help us to lose weight and gain muscle, it is also proven to reduce stress and elevate mood. Exercise also helps us burn fat *and* build muscle. Combined with the anti-inflammatory diet this is the ideal combination for success.

Physical exercise has wonderful anti-inflammatory effects. No one kind of exercise is better than another; ideally you have a range of activities that incorporate aerobics, weight training, and flexibility exercises such as stretching, yoga, or Pilates. The key is that exercise really does need to be performed on a regular basis to confer optimal benefits. In this chapter you will find a wide variety of guidelines and helpful tips to help you construct a customized exercise plan, based on your personal needs and capabilities.

In an ideal world, we would exercise at least five times per week for 30–45 minutes per day. For many of us, it is helpful to exercise Monday through Friday either before or after work. We can then give ourselves the weekends off. This can be an effective plan since we tend to be active on weekends, running errands and performing other physical chores–as opposed to the desk jobs that many of us are tied to during the week. But if the Monday through Friday routine seems just too daunting a task, remember that every little bit helps. If three times per week is more doable, then start with that. If you can exercise in only 10-minute increments three to five times a day, that helps too! But, don't try to make up for a week of inactivity by overdoing it on the weekend. Overexercising or spending long grueling hours at some so-called leisure activity is pro-inflammatory–limit your exercise session to no more than 45 minutes.

Overexercising can trigger the release of the stress hormone cortisol, which can cause unwanted weight gain (especially in the abdominal area–more about this dangerous form of fat in Chapter 8), break down muscle tissue, and accelerate the rate at which we age (more about this later).

In addition to increasing your overall physical health, regular exercise will greatly assist any weight-loss or weight-maintenance program. But perhaps best of all is the feeling of satisfaction, self-esteem, and accomplishment that you will have when you have a regular exercise routine–and stick to it. Truthfully, this is one of the only things we do that is for our benefit and ours alone; the rest of our day is spent in the service of trying to please our boss, spouse, family, and friends. Exercise is also great for the skin, giving you a radiant glow that no amount of makeup can duplicate!

WHAT YOU NEED IS A PLAN

An interesting study conducted at the University of Alberta and published in the journal *Psychology of Sport and Exercise* reported that the exercise strategy that really works is a simple one: "Just Do It"–those three little words made famous by Nike. The study reports that people who are successful at exercising regularly don't stop to think about it; they really do "just do it," according to Dr. Sandra Cousins, professor of physical education and recreation at the University of Alberta.

In-depth interviews with 40 Alberta men and women aged 42 to 77 revealed that those who exercise regularly don't employ pep talks or think much about the pros or cons of participating.

"We used to think that positive self-talk was important to promote individual exercise participation, but when it comes to the general public, you don't need a pep talk," said Dr. Cousins.

Here are three foolproof ways to ensure that you exercise regularly:

1. Build a solid routine that you follow faithfully–let nothing get in its way. Schedule exercise for a realistic time. You already know if 6:00 A.M. is too early for you to get up and take a walk or if you're too tired to go to the gym at 6:00 P.M. when you get off of work.

2. Find an exercise partner and a set routine that you share; this will keep you both motivated and you will have fun together.

3. Find activities you genuinely enjoy. Don't start running if you hate solitary endurance exercises. Think creatively. Remember what you liked to do as a kid or think of something you've always wanted to learn. Take ice skating or roller blading lessons. Play tennis with your son or daughter. Go to dance classes. Start swimming. Get a bike–bikes today have amazing gearing systems making even steep hills easy to climb. Get a dog and take long walks together. There are truly lots of possibilities.

The aerobic part of my routine, for example, is to run on the treadmill every morning before I begin my day. This is the first thing I do after getting out of bed. If I wait until later, 1,001 excuses, interruptions, and distractions will get in the way, and

I will not get to exercise. I also find that I have increased energy throughout the day thanks to the exercise, and an elevated mood as well. When I don't exercise, I am more easily fatigued, both mentally and physically.

Some of the best exercise guidelines I've seen and am sharing with you come from the President's Council on Physical Fitness (PCPFS) www.fitness.gov. Use this website freely and often. It contains a wealth of valuable information geared to helping us achieve physical fitness and a healthy lifestyle—regardless of age.

GET MOVING, GET BREATHING

According to the PCPFS, although any kind of physical movement requires energy (calories), the type of exercise that uses the most energy is aerobic exercise. The term "aerobic" is derived from the Greek word meaning "with oxygen." In exercise circles, it is used to describe any exercise that increases the need for oxygen. Aerobic exercise causes your heart to beat harder and faster, carrying more oxygen to your hard-at-work muscles, which then use oxygen to convert glucose and fat into energy. Jogging, brisk walking, swimming, biking, skating, cross-country skiing, and dancing are some popular forms of aerobic exercise.

Aerobic exercises use the body's large muscle groups in continuous, rhythmic, sustained movement and require oxygen for the production of energy. When oxygen is combined with food (which can come from stored fat) energy is produced to power the body's musculature. The longer you move aerobically, the more energy is needed and the more calories used—just remember that strenuous workouts such as running and aerobic dancing should be limited to 45 minutes. Regular aerobic exercise will improve the ability of your heart, lungs, blood vessels, and associated tissues to use oxygen to produce energy needed for activity. You'll build a healthier body while getting rid of excess body fat.

HOW MUCH? HOW OFTEN?

Experts recommend that you do some form of aerobic exercise at least three times a week for a minimum of 20 to 30 continuous minutes. As you build up your strength and endurance, strive to extend this to a maximum of 45 minutes; remember overexertion is inflammatory. Of course, if that is too much, start with a shorter time span and gradually build up to the maximum. If you need to lose a large amount of weight, you may want to do your aerobic workout five times a week.

It is important to exercise at an intensity vigorous enough to cause your heart rate and breathing to increase. How hard you should exercise depends to a certain degree on your age and is determined by measuring your heart rate in beats per minute.

The heart rate you should maintain is called your "target heart rate," and there are several ways you can arrive at this figure. The simplest is to subtract your age from 220 and then calculate 60 to 80 percent of that figure. Beginners should maintain the 60 percent level, more advanced can work up to the 80 percent level. This is just a guide, however, and people with any medical limitations should discuss this formula with their physician.

You can do different types of aerobic activities, say walking one day, riding a bike the next. Make sure you choose an activity that can be done regularly and is enjoyable for you. The important thing to remember is not to skip too many days between workouts or fitness benefits will be lost. If you must lose a few days, gradually work back into your routine.

PHYSICAL ACTIVITY FACT SHEET
(CITATION: U.S. DEPARTMENT OF HEALTH
AND HUMAN SERVICES)

Physical inactivity, combined with poor eating habits, contributes to 300,000 preventable deaths a year in the United States. More than 40 percent of deaths in the United States are caused by behavior patterns that could be modified. A sedentary lifestyle is a major risk factor across the spectrum of preventable diseases that lower the quality of life and kill Americans. Poor diet and physical inactivity (combined) are rapidly approaching tobacco (435,000 deaths) as the leading cause of preventable death in the United States.

◆ Adults 18 and older need 30 minutes of physical activity on five or more days a week to be healthy; children and teens need 60 minutes of activity a day for their health.

▼

- Significant health benefits can be obtained by including a moderate amount of physical activity (e.g., 30 minutes of brisk walking or raking leaves, 15 minutes of running, 45 minutes of playing volleyball). Additional health benefits can be gained through greater amounts of physical activity.

▼

- Thirty to sixty minutes of activity broken into smaller segments of 10 or 15 minutes throughout the day has significant health benefits but remember the guidelines above and limit longer sessions to 45 minutes.

▼

- Moderate daily physical activity can reduce substantially the risk of developing or dying from cardiovascular disease, type 2 diabetes, and certain cancers, such as colon cancer. Daily physical activity helps to lower blood pressure and cholesterol, helps prevent or retard osteoporosis, and helps reduce obesity, symptoms of anxiety and depression, and symptoms of arthritis.

▼

- Cardiovascular disease (heart attacks, strokes) is the number one killer of men and women in the United States. Physically inactive people are twice as likely to develop coronary heart disease as regularly active people. The health risk posed by physical inactivity is almost as high as risk factors such as cigarette smoking, high blood pressure, and high cholesterol.

ENERGY EXPENDITURE CHART

On the following page is a chart that delineates how many calories we burn in an hour performing various activities. Although I don't focus on counting calories in the Perricone Weight-Loss Diet, they can be a useful way of figuring out how hard your body is working. Just adding 15 minutes of moderate exercise, for example, to your daily schedule will begin to have a noticeable effect on your health and appearance.

Also on the PCPFS site is the Nolan Ryan Fitness Guide, which contains excellent information on stretching for flexibility, reprinted on the next page:

Energy Expenditure Chart

A. Sedentary Activities	Energy Costs Cals/Hour*
Lying down or sleeping	90
Sitting quietly	84
Sitting and writing, card playing, etc.	114

B. Moderate Activities	(150–350)
Bicycling (5 mph)	174
Canoeing (2.5 mph)	174
Dancing (ballroom)	210
Golf (2-some, carrying clubs)	324
Horseback riding (sitting to trot)	246
Light housework, cleaning, etc.	246
Swimming (crawl, 20 yards/min)	288
Tennis (recreational doubles)	312
Volleyball (recreational)	264
Walking (2 mph)	198

C. Vigorous Activities	More than 350
Aerobic dancing	546
Basketball (recreational)	450
Bicycling (13 mph)	612
Circuit weight training	756
Football (touch, vigorous)	498
Ice skating (9 mph)	384
Racquetball	588
Roller skating (9 mph)	384
Jogging (10 minute mile, 6 mph)	654
Scrubbing floors	440
Swimming (crawl, 45 yards/min)	522
Tennis (recreational singles)	450
X-country skiing (5 mph)	690

*Hourly estimates based on values calculated for calories burned per minute for a 150-pound (68 kg) person.

STRETCHING: REACH FOR FLEXIBILITY

Stretching, though often overlooked, plays a vital role in keeping muscles and joints strong and pliable so they are less susceptible to injury. That's why it is such an important part of warming up before physical activity and cooling down after.

Spending a few minutes a day doing slow, deliberate stretches can also help you manage stress more effectively. It will give you a chance to momentarily shut off outside stressors, and focus, physically and mentally, on your activity, and it will physically help to relax your muscles. Try just 5 to 10 minutes of gentle stretching when you come home from work at night and see how much calmer you will feel. You'll be amazed to find how much tension you were carrying around in your body.

Books and articles describing specific stretches abound. A good routine should work each of the major muscle groups, and needn't take long. Five to 10 minutes is all you need. Be sure to scan the Rules to Stretch By before you begin.

RULES TO STRETCH BY

- Warm up first: warm muscles, tendons, and ligaments are more flexible and stretch more easily; stretching cold muscles can cause tears.
- Stretches should always be gradual and gentle.
- Hold each stretch in a static position for 10 to 20 seconds, allowing the muscle to lengthen slowly.
- Do not bounce; bouncing actually causes muscle fibers to shorten, not lengthen.
- Stretch only to the point of resistance; if the stretch hurts, you're pushing too hard.
- Don't rush through the stretching routine; use it to prepare yourself mentally and physically for activity.

STRENGTH AND RESISTANCE TRAINING

The National Institute of Aging has a website (www.niapublications.org) that is an outstanding resource on all forms of exercises and even includes drawings and animations of actual exercises in the following categories.

1. Resistance
2. Endurance
3. Balance
4. Stretching

Strength exercises are designed to improve muscle mass and to strengthen bone. According to the NIA, even very small changes in muscle size can make a big difference in strength, especially in people who already have lost a lot of muscle. An increase in muscle that's not even visible to the eye can be all it takes to improve your ability to do things like get up from a chair or climb stairs.

Strength exercises require you to lift or push weights and gradually increase the amount of weight you use. You can use the hand and ankle weights sold in sporting-goods stores and chain stores such as Kmart and Wal-Mart. They are inexpensive and indestructible, providing years of service.

You can also buy a resistance band (it looks like a giant rubber band, and stretching it helps build muscle) at a sporting-goods store to do other types of strength exercises. Or you can use the special strength-training equipment at a fitness center.

HOW MUCH, HOW OFTEN

◆ Do strength exercises for all of your major muscle groups **at least twice a week.** Don't do strength exercises of the same muscle group on any 2 days in a row.

▼

◆ Depending on your condition, you might need to start out using as little as 1 or 2 pounds of weight, or no weight at all. The tissues that bind the structures of your body together need to adapt to strength exercises.

▼

◆ **Use a minimum of weight the first week,** then gradually add weight. Starting out with weights that are too heavy can cause injuries.

▼

◆ Gradually add a challenging amount of weight in order to benefit from strength exercises. If you don't challenge your muscles, you won't benefit from strength exercises.

▼

◆ When doing a strength exercise, do **8 to 15 repetitions in a row.** Wait a minute, then do another set of 8 to 15 repetitions in a row of the same exercise. (Tip: While you are waiting, you might want to stretch the muscle you just worked or do a different strength exercise that uses a different set of muscles.)

▼

◆ Take **3 seconds to lift or push a weight** into place; **hold the position for 1 second,** and take **another 3 seconds to lower the weight.** Don't let the weight drop; lowering it slowly is very important.

▼

- It should feel somewhere between hard and very hard for you to lift or push the weight. It should not feel very, very hard. If you can't lift or push a weight 8 times in a row, it's too heavy for you. Reduce the amount of weight. If you can lift a weight more than 15 times in a row, it's too light for you. Increase the amount of weight.

▼

- Stretch after strength exercises, when your muscles are warmed up. If you stretch before strength exercises, be sure to warm up your muscles first (through light walking and arm pumping, for example).

SAFETY TIPS FOR STRENGTH TRAINING

- **Don't hold your breath during strength exercises.** Breathe normally. Holding your breath while straining can cause changes in blood pressure. This is especially true for people with cardiovascular disease.

▼

- If you have had a hip or knee repair or replacement, check with your surgeon before doing lower-body exercises.

▼

- Avoid jerking or thrusting weights into position. That can cause injuries. Use smooth, steady movements.

▼

- Avoid "locking" the joints in your arms and legs in a tightly straightened position. (A tip on how to straighten your knees: Tighten your thigh muscles. This will lift your kneecaps and protect them.)

▼

- Breathe out as you lift or push, and breathe in as you relax. For example, if you are doing leg lifts, breathe out as you lift your leg, and breathe in as you lower it. This may not feel natural at first, and you probably will have to think about it as you are doing it for a while.

▼

- Muscle soreness lasting up to a few days and slight fatigue are normal after muscle-building exercises, but exhaustion, sore joints, and unpleasant muscle pulling aren't. The latter symptoms mean you are overdoing it.

- None of the exercises you do should cause pain. The range within which you move your arms and legs should never hurt.

PROGRESSING

- Gradually increasing the amount of weight you use is crucial for building strength.

  ▼

- When you are able to lift a weight between 8 and 15 times, you can increase the amount of weight you use at your next session.

  ▼

- Here is an example of how to progress gradually: Start out with a weight that you can lift only 8 times. Keep using that weight until you become strong enough to lift it 12 to 15 times. Add more weight so that, again, you can lift it only 8 times. Use this weight until you can lift it 12 to 15 times, then add more weight. Keep repeating.

  For more information, visit www.niapublications.org

TIPS TO GET YOU STARTED AND KEEP YOU GOING

I hope by now I've convinced you that you will be healthier and happier if you include exercise in your daily routine. It's a change worth making. Here are some tips, courtesy of the PCSPF, to get you started:

1. Check with your doctor first. It is wise to get your doctor's OK before embarking on an exercise program, especially if you are carrying around some extra "baggage."

2. Set short-term goals that aren't related to your weight. It helps to see exercise as

something of value for its own sake. Keep a record of your progress and tell your friends and family about your achievements.

3. Adopt a specific plan and write it down.

4. Keep setting realistic goals as you go along, and remind yourself of them often.

5. Keep a log to record your progress and make sure to keep it up to date.

6. Include weight and/or percent body fat measures in your log.

7. Upgrade your fitness program as you progress.

8. Enlist the support and company of your family and friends.

9. Update others on your successes.

10. Avoid injuries by pacing yourself and include a warm-up and cool-down period as part of every workout.

11. Reward yourself periodically for a job well done!

STRESS, STRESS-RELATED WEIGHT GAIN, AND OBESITY

Stress is highly destructive—not just emotionally, but also physically. Unfortunately, in today's world, we all experience significant amounts of stress, and it does not appear to be going away anytime soon.

Many circumstances create stress in our daily lives. Arguing with family, friends, or colleagues, not getting enough sleep, worrying about everything from our family to our finances, constant pressure to keep up with the home and office demands; even playing too hard can all create stress. Weekend warriors, making up for a week of inactivity by spending hours engaged in strenuous activity, are also setting themselves up for a stress response.

CORTISOL, THE STRESS/DEATH HORMONE

When we are under stress, our adrenal glands produce hormones. These include the fight-or-flight hormones, epinephrine (adrenaline) and norepinephrine (noradrenaline), as well as cortisol.

Cortisol is a glucocorticoid, one of a group of steroid hormones that include cortisone. Cortisol is involved in carbohydrate, protein, and fat metabolism, and has anti-inflammatory properties. As we age, the "youth" hormones such as testosterone, estrogen, and human growth hormone decline. Cortisol, however, increases as we age and too much cortisol can also become pro-inflammatory.

When we experience stress (whether from fear, anxiety, physical or emotional trauma, or overexertion), the stress hormones epinephrine and norepinephrine will return to normal levels as the stress subsides. In a young person, cortisol levels will also return to normal within a few hours. Because cortisol levels continue to rise with age, the older person's cortisol levels will remain elevated for long periods of time. This has earned cortisol the dubious distinction of being known as a "death" hormone, because high levels of cortisol exert a catabolic or muscle-wasting, deteriorating action on the body. Simply put, it breaks down tissue.

HOW STRESS PROMOTES WEIGHT GAIN

Cortisol stimulates fat and carbohydrate metabolism for fast energy (the fight-or-flight response), thereby stimulating insulin release to keep pace with the rising blood sugar levels. This results in an increase in our appetite. If we experience chronic stress, with chronically high levels of cortisol, we may end up hungry all the time, causing us to overeat.

Cortisol also influences where that weight will be deposited. A fascinating study on the effects of the release of cortisol during acute and chronic stress in nonoverweight women was published in the journal *Psychosomatic Medicine* in 2001. The study clearly demonstrated that this excess cortisol contributes to the deposition of visceral fat, particularly in the abdominal region. As we know, there are two types of fat: subcutaneous (under the skin) and visceral (found in the abdomen and surrounding our vital organs). In Hope's story in Chapter 8, her fat was centered in the abdomen (also termed "central obesity"). Although Hope was not seriously overweight, she had excess fat around the waist and it showed.

Central obesity sets the stage for a host of health concerns such as heart disease, strokes, and diabetes. Because of its serious threat to health, this has also been referred to as "toxic fat." Traditionally, women worried about the size of their hips. However, when it comes to overall weight gain, it is preferable to have it on the hips as opposed to the stomach area—if not from an aesthetic point of view, then from a health point of view. Studies indicate that women (and men) who store their weight in the abdominal area have higher cortisol levels and higher stress levels than those whose weight is stored on the hips.

THE CHOLESTEROL COMPONENT

In addition, visceral fat is metabolized by the liver, which turns it into cholesterol that circulates in the blood. This is the so-called "bad" cholesterol, low-density lipoproteins or LDL, which collects in the arteries forming plaque (deposits of fats, inflammatory cells, proteins, and calcium material along the lining of arteries). The plaque builds up and narrows the artery, resulting in atherosclerosis. Researchers have also found that consuming a lot of saturated fats such as butter and the fats found in red meats can lead to the accumulation of visceral fat. The high omega-3 content found in wild Alaskan salmon, anchovies, sardines, and other cold-water fish, along with fish oil capsules will help you to get rid of this deadly form of fat because the essential fatty acids found in these foods can decrease cortisol levels.

To sum up, elevated cortisol levels produce a host of negative effects that include

- increased inflammation
- increased insulin secretion
- increased appetite
- storage of fat, particularly in the abdomen
- increased risk of acne flareups. Acne is a systemic inflammatory disease and stress precipitates and aggravates acne breakouts.
- the death of brain cells. High levels of stress actually shrink the brain and other organs.
- destruction of the immune system
- decreased muscle mass
- accelerated aging

In addition, a cortisol excess can lead to a progressive loss of protein, and collagen is the most abundant protein in the human body. This results in the progressive thinning and reduction in collagen of the tissue—including the skin—caused mainly by an inhibited collagen synthesis. Remember, excess collagen is "catabolic," that is, it breaks down tissue. It removes the protein from the skin, for example, and shuttles it into the muscle to prepare the body for the fight-or-flight adrenal response (cortisol is an adrenal hormone). This thinner skin takes on a more translucent appearance resulting in prominent blood vessels and visible veins.

LOWER STRESS LEVELS TO SLIM DOWN AND SHAPE UP

In addition to regular, moderate exercise, there are a variety of stress-reducing activities that are easy to do and, for the most part, free:

- **Quiet Contemplation:** Prayer, meditation, or yoga; taking walks in the park, along the beach or in the forest; reading a good book; and spending time with good friends have proven benefits. Research by Paul Ekman of the University of California San Francisco Medical Center suggests that meditation and mindfulness can tame the amygdala, an area of the brain that is the hub of fear memory. Scientists working in the field of neuroplasticity have discovered that how we focus our attention over time can change the actual biology of our brains, which is one reason to avoid watching television. Much of what is on television is aimed at raising your cortisol levels—whether it is the stress of the courtroom, the ER, the ubiquitous scenes of gratuitous violence and victimization, the evening news, or even watching your favorite sports team get trounced. If you are concerned about your weight, consider this fact. Those known for spending hours in front of the TV are known as "couch potatoes," and I have yet to hear anyone ever referred to as a "couch stringbean."

▼

- **The Healing Power of Pets:** Normal day-to-day interactions with our partners and children can be stressful, no matter how much we love them. I've said this in my other books, but I can't say it often enough: one of my favorite, all-time ways to relieve stress is to spend time with my dog. Not only does he make me laugh with his spunky personality and antics, his unstinting devotion and loyalty are always heartwarming and validating. Hundreds of studies have proven beyond a doubt that owning a loving, nonjudgmental companion animal is good for you, mentally, physically, and emotionally. The simple stroking of a dog or cat has been proven to lower heart rate, decrease stress and anxiety, and lower respiratory rate and blood pressure. Even watching fish in an aquarium creates similar effects. It is both soothing and meditative. With our stress and obesity levels at an all-time high, we just might save two lives when we adopt a loving pet from the local shelter—theirs and ours.

▼

- **Laugh to Lose Weight:** We need to implement stress reducing strategies not only to lose weight but for our overall health, because as we can see, chronic high levels of stress are no laughing matter. But laughter is an excellent antidote to stress. We have all heard the old saying "Laughter is the best medicine." As is often the case, these time-honored aphorisms hold more than a kernel of truth. There is very strong evidence that laughter can actually improve health and help fight disease. In 1989, researchers at Loma Linda University School of Medicine did a study demonstrating that laughter reduces epinephrine, cortisol, dopamine, and growth hormone, four of the neuroendocrine hormones associated with the stress response. They also discovered that laughter played a significant role in strengthening the immune system, lowering blood pressure, acting as a muscle relaxant, triggering the release of endorphins (the body's natural painkillers), and producing a general sense of well-being.

▼

- **Take Time for Tea:** Other than water, tea is the most widely consumed beverage in the world. There are many varieties of tea and they all possess healthful properties. For our purposes we are going to focus on the most popular forms of tea, best known for their superior antioxidant ability. These are white, black, and green tea.

  1. **White Tea**—a Chinese tea whose unfermented leaves are amber, and only the tips of the tea plant are used. A recent study on white tea confirmed the following: the antiviral and antibacterial effect of white tea (Stash and Templar brands) is greater than that of green tea; the antiviral and antibacterial effect of several toothpastes including Aim, Aquafresh, Colgate, Crest, and Orajel was enhanced by the addition of white tea extract; white tea extract exhibited an antifungal effect on both *Penicillium chrysogenum* and *Saccharomyces cerevisiae;* and white tea extract may have application in the inactivation of pathogenic human microbes, i.e., bacteria, viruses, and fungi.

  2. **Black Tea**—made of green tea leaves that have been oxidized, or fermented,

What's in a Cup of Tea*

Substance	Special points
Catechins	More than half of the total catechin content is epigallocatechin gallate, which is also known as EGCG. It is 20 times more powerful than vitamin C as an antioxidant.
Thearubigins	A complex flavonoid that develops when leaves of tea are fermented and turn black.
Theaflavins	Also produced during fermentation of the leaves.
Caffeine	Mild stimulant found in tea, a 200 ml cup contains an average of 40 mg of caffeine compared to 64 mg in instant coffee and up to 150 mg in brewed coffee (green tea and white tea have even less caffeine).
Tannin	A type of flavonoid that adds flavor, astringency, and bitterness to tea, in addition to its antioxidant properties.

* The European Food Information Council (www.eufic.org).

and imparting a characteristic reddish brew, is far and away the most widely consumed tea—especially in the United States. Black tea is cardioprotective, has anticancer properties, boosts the body's natural defenses, improves blood flow to coronary arteries, and helps speed recovery after heart attack.

The plant nutrients in tea are called "flavonoids", an integral part of the plant world that provide important antioxidant functions. They help deactivate free radicals and decrease harmful inflammation. Just one cup of tea supplies around 200 mg of flavonoids, many of which are released into the drink within the first minute of brewing. To learn more about the health benefits of tea, visit the European Food Information Council (www.eufic.org) a nonprofit educational organization.

3. **Green Tea**—originates in China, Japan, and other parts of Asia. It is made from the fresh leaves of the tea plant that are steamed, rolled, and dried at high temperatures. Because it has important implications in weight loss, it re-

ceives the most extensive coverage of the tea family in the Perricone Weight-Loss Diet.

Studies have shown the thermogenic and fat oxidation properties of green tea and have proven that green tea prevents the absorption of fat, helping to keep excess body fat under control. An even newer study appeared in the *Annals of Nutrition & Metabolism,* 2005, showing for the first time that supplementation with the most plentiful green tea polyphenol, EGCG, abolishes–actually stops–diet-induced obesity. According to the study, this effect is at least partly caused by the EGCG exerting a direct influence on adipose tissue. The study concluded: "Dietary supplementation with EGCG should be considered as a valuable natural treatment option for obesity."

A recent study in the United Kingdom found that chemicals in the tea also shut down a key molecule that can play a significant role in the development of cancer. Green tea has been credited with helping a variety of health conditions including arthritis, lowered blood sugar levels, and lowered blood pressure. Always choose organic.

▼

◆ **Clock Work:** As we discussed in the exercise portion of this chapter, we need a steady fixed routine for an exercise program to succeed. We humans are creatures of habits–for better or worse. We like to eat our meals at the same time, go to bed at the same time, and so on.

It turns out that there is an excellent reason for this. We all need to follow a daily circadian rhythm–that is, a rhythm based on the 24-hour cycle. For thousands of years this was not a problem. Humans went to sleep when the sun went down and arose when the sun came up. However, those days are long gone. And it appears that this is not a positive change, as scientists have discovered that disruption of this cycle causes us to develop a series of metabolic discords.

Staying up too late, snacking throughout the day, and skipping meals, all upset the genes that control daily rhythms in the brain and throughout the body. One important study found that the "clock," which scientists thought was only in the central part of the brain, is also present in the part of the brain that controls appetite.

It now appears that biological clocks function not only in the brain but in many parts of the body as well. They govern not only the sleep cycle but also functions including fluid balance, body temperature, oxygen consumption—and now, it has been shown, appetite. According to one of the lead researchers, Dr. Joseph Bass, the finding offers no immediate solution to the human problem of obesity or related health problems such as diabetes. However, he believes that it adds to the abundant evidence that timing is important in eating habits. It appears that synchronization of mealtimes has a direct impact on our weight.

Another member of the research team stated that the study provided new genetic evidence that physiological outputs of the biological clock, like sleep and appetite, are interconnected at the molecular and behavioral levels. Perhaps more important, it establishes the fact that we need to follow a regimen in our daily lives, one based on cycles that we have been acclimated to since the dawn of time, such as the rising and setting of the sun. While it is not practical to go to bed with the sun, it does make sense to get up with it, and this provides us with a good excuse to not stay up to all hours and become sleep deprived—another startling cause of increased appetite, carbohydrate craving, and unwanted weight gain.

Ideally we will follow a regular routine, which means going to bed at the same time each night, arising at the same time each morning, and following a regular pattern for our mealtimes. We need to keep our bodies on a schedule in the same way we keep other areas of our lives on schedule. If you have ever been a parent, you know how important a steady routine is for the well-being of your children, especially when they're babies. We all know what happens when that schedule becomes upset! So feel free to "baby" yourself; you will feel healthier and happier and be much less likely to overeat.

▼

♦ **Sleep to Lose Weight:** An important study at the University of Chicago demonstrated that sleep deprivation causes us to overeat. When we don't get enough sleep, our levels of ghrelin, a hormone produced by stomach cells and believed to increase feelings of hunger, increase. Leptin, a hormone produced by our fat cells that suppresses appetite and burns fat stores, is decreased. It is easy to see how this can add to overeating and weight gain. In addition, the people in the study who were the most sleep deprived craved carbohydrate-rich (i.e., the most fattening!) foods, such as sweets, pasta, and breads. According to the lead researcher of the study, Eve Van Cauter, Ph.D., levels of cortisol were also higher during sleep deprivation periods than when the study subjects were fully rested. They also metabolized glucose less efficiently. Dr. Van Cauter reported that the effects of sleep deprivation on glucose metabolism were similar to those found in the elderly. She therefore concluded that chronic sleep deprivation may have long-term harmful effects on the body—not the least of which is weight gain and possible accelerated aging as well.

▼

◆ **Water Wisdom:** Logic tells us that when we have an unwanted fire, we throw water on it to put it out. Therefore it makes perfect sense that water would help quell the cellular inflammation that goes on in our bodies. In fact, this is true. Water *will* decrease inflammation in the body.

Approximately 65 to 70 percent of the body weight is water. Water maintains moisture in the body; it transports oxygen to the blood and helps carry nutrients through blood. Water is necessary to maintain an ideal internal body temperature—in fact, nearly every biological function requires the help of water.

Water naturally suppresses the appetite and helps the body metabolize stored fat. Studies have shown that if we decrease our water intake our fat deposits will increase. Conversely, an increase in water intake will reduce fat deposits. One of the roles of our liver is to convert stored fat to energy. Because our kidneys can't function properly without enough water, if we don't have enough water in our systems, the liver steps in and assists kidney function. This results in the liver not being able to metabolize fats as quickly and efficiently as it did when it was not assisting the kidneys. As a result, it metabolizes less fat; more fat remains stored in the body and weight loss stops.

Water is essential to fat metabolism. The more you weigh, the more water you need. An even mildly dehydrated body will cause a 3 percent drop in baseline metabolism resulting in the gain of one pound of fat every six months. A dehydrated body will also provoke the development of aging, inflammatory compounds. Dehydration is also a major cause of fatigue.

When we give our bodies adequate water (six to eight 8-ounce glasses per day—or approximately two quarts), we should notice a decrease in our appetites. Women and body builders have often avoided drinking enough water because they fear bloating. You will not become bloated; in fact, the opposite will occur: the well-defined look will be enhanced as more fat is metabolized and wastes are flushed from the body.

As we can see, gaining unwanted weight has a variety of simple pro-inflammatory causes and just as simple anti-inflammatory remedies:

- follow the anti-inflammatory diet
- follow a regular (ideally daily) exercise regimen
- get enough sleep
- don't skip meals
- don't snack all day
- stay well hydrated
- learn how to control stress

The next section of the book contains the actual 14-day plan. Follow the many tips on foods to look for and foods to avoid in Chapter 8, and the 14-day plan in Chapter 9, and in just two weeks, you will have embarked on a way of living that will not only help you lose weight and keep your weight down, it will also keep you healthier and happier for the rest of your life.

PART III

The Plan

Chapter 8

Important Tips to Remember on the 14-Day Perricone Weight-Loss Diet

After thirty, a body has a mind of its own.
— Bette Midler

If you have found yourself echoing the same sentiments as Bette—don't despair. The 14-day Weight-Loss Diet provides you with multiple strategies that will trick your body into forgetting the passage of the years!

The story of Hope is a great case in point and the finest way I can think of to introduce the 14-Day Perricone Weight-Loss Diet. Millions of people first met Hope when she appeared with me on *Oprah*—she was there to show the effects that the Perricone Program had on her skin. The audience was speechless at how radiant and wonderful she looked when viewing her "before" photo and then seeing her "after" in person.

However, there was another side to the story. Hope had experienced a dramatic weight loss and a great increase in overall health, vitality, and energy, as well as the rejuvenated complexion.

Although a weight of 133 on a frame of 5 feet 7 might seem like a dream to many of us, Hope's weight had settled around the lower half of her body, especially in the abdomen area. This can mean that she was storing the type of fat we call "visceral." Visceral fat is of greater concern than the more common subcutaneous fat that lies just below the skin. This fat surrounds vital organs and is metabolized by the liver, which turns it into blood cholesterol. People who consume large amounts of saturated fat and people who perform little or no physical activity are likely to have high stores

Hope's Story

Hope started the Perricone Program during a very taxing time in her life, dealing with the sudden onset of difficult health and emotional issues. Instead of crumbling under the stress, Hope, who had always been fascinated by the link between food and good health, decided to give the Perricone Program a try. She read my books and learned how a diet filled with inflammatory foods exacerbates many diseases. Hope was convinced—wasn't her current health problem indicative of what can happen when the bulk of your diet consists of greasy take-out and starch-laden "comfort" foods?

After just a few days of focusing solely on the foods that have powerful anti-inflammatory properties, Hope saw and felt incredible results, inspiring her to introduce this new way of eating to both her husband and 11-month-old son.

"I used to feel sick after every meal," Hope confessed. "I have always had a really weak stomach. I always felt heavy. I never really noticed until after I started following Dr. Perricone's approach, just how dragged down I had felt before. I'd eat something and it felt like it would just sit in my stomach."

Those weren't the only adverse effects Hope experienced.

"My body was scarred and flabby," she admits. "My face was damaged from the sun . . . it was inflamed and red. I suffered from breakouts and creeping wrinkles."

Hope switched from coffee to green tea and lots of pure water. She cut back on a lot of red meat and introduced fresh fish—especially wild Alaskan salmon. Processed, sugary, and starchy foods were eliminated and replaced with nourishing choices such as old-fashioned oatmeal, fresh fruits and vegetables, plain yogurt, and raw unsalted nuts and seeds.

"I ate breakfast that first morning and loved it," Hope recalls.

"My energy level after the first meal evened out. I felt amazing. I asked my husband, John, if he, too, noticed a difference, and he said he'd never felt like this before. We couldn't believe it. Nobody had ever taught us how to eat right."

Hope soon lost 10 pounds while John lost 12. And after only three days, the redness and puffiness in her face began to diminish. After four weeks on the program Hope looked and felt like a new person. When her "before" photograph was shown on the TV monitor at the Oprah show, the audience saw a slightly overweight young woman with a red, blotchy complexion. An audible, collective gasp arose from the audience as the video camera zoomed in for a live shot of Hope in the audience. Her peaches and cream complexion glowed with vibrant beauty and health. Gone were all traces of redness and puffiness. Her body looked lean and fit. Truthfully, the audience could not believe that such a change could be effected by diet alone.

But Hope was and is living proof of the power of the anti-inflammatory lifestyle.

of visceral fat. While Hope was not the proverbial couch potato, she did eat a lot of junk food, trans fats, and saturated fats.

By following the Perricone anti-inflammatory diet, Hope lost ten pounds—and the good news is that she lost fat and not muscle. Her remarkable physical and mental transformation that captured the imagination of *Oprah* viewers worldwide helped encourage me to write this book.

Hope's story is but one of a great many similar stories detailing success with the Perricone Program—all inspiring and all empowering.

BEFORE YOU START THE PERRICONE WEIGHT-LOSS DIET

Keep these three tips in mind for the best results from the 14-day program:

1. Remember, every meal or snack must include: protein, low-glycemic carbs, essential fatty acids.

2. Always eat your protein first. Reach for that shrimp cocktail or smoked salmon appetizer first—and when your Thanksgiving dinner entrée arrives, eat the turkey first, followed by your green salad and vegetables. Why? Because by eating your protein first at every meal you are helping to suppress your appetite. Proteins are digested much more slowly than carbohydrates—even carbohydrates that are high in fiber. Also protein is neutral in terms of its effect on blood sugar.

3. Save the fresh fruit for the end of the meal. This way, you will prevent the natural sugars found in the fruit from causing a spike in blood sugar. Our goal is to avoid spikes in blood sugar, which trigger insulin release. Remember this fact: insulin release = stored fat!

FISH FACTS

Fish is very important in the anti-inflammatory weight-loss diet. Many people think that they "hate" fish—particularly salmon. However, when you understand what an amazing weight-loss food salmon is (as well as a fat-burner, muscle-builder, wrinkle-eraser, skin-saver, depression-lifter, and brain-booster) you may want to reconsider and give it a chance. Sometimes it may simply be that you have not had the *right* piece of salmon (check the Resource Guide for salmon that will forever change the way you think about this miracle food!). In an ideal world, you will enjoy four to five fish meals per week. I personally have even more than that. And give some of the simple yet delightful recipes in Chapter 9 a try—you just might be very pleasantly surprised.

- Avoid farm raised salmon—wild Alaskan salmon is superior in every way. Canned salmon is almost always wild Alaskan salmon (read the label) and can be used in salads, to make delicious salmon burgers, soups, and chowders, and so on.

▼

- Introduce anchovies, herring, and sardines into your diet. Like wild Alaskan salmon, these tiny little fish will really ramp up your ability to shed fat! And like wild Alaskan salmon, they are rich sources of the omega-3 essential fatty acids. Anchovies can be mashed and added to sauces and salad dressing—the classic Caesar salad dressing owes its unique, incomparable flavor to the addition of anchovy paste or a few mashed anchovies. If you want to help your skin stay taut and toned on face and body, eat liberal amounts of these miracle fish. In addition to omega-3s, they contain DMAE, which helps ensure adequate levels of the neurotransmitters that contribute to the maintenance of muscle tone on face and body. Serve them on crackers made out of flaxseed and Bragg's Amino Acid liquid for a delicious snack or lunch treat—just add an apple and a bottle of water! (See the Resource Guide to learn more about this delicious alternative to traditional crackers.)

OPT FOR ORGANIC FOR THE CHICKEN, THE EGG, AND THE DAIRY

- Whenever possible, select organic, free range chicken and turkey. For optimum health and weight management avoid the antibiotics, hormones, and processing of regular commercially raised poultry.

▼

◆ Thanks to the wonderful addition of flaxseed to the diet of chickens, we can now purchase eggs from cage-free chickens that are fed diets of flaxseeds, making these eggs good sources of omega-3s. They are now widely available in regular supermarkets and are a much healthier choice than conventional eggs.

▼

◆ When choosing dairy products, look for organic brands whose cows are raised without antibiotics or hormones. Read labels and avoid products containing preservatives such as postassium sorbate, fillers, stabilizers, guar gum, carageenan, and other unnecessary, unpronounceable ingredients! The label for cottage cheese, for example, should list only the following ingredients: cultured pasteurized Grade A skim milk, milk, cream, and salt.

FRUITS AND VEGETABLES—RICH SOURCES OF ANTI-INFLAMMATORY PHYTONUTRIENTS AND FIBER

◆ Choose organic fruits and vegetables when possible. Pesticides can leave toxic residues on plants that can harm your organ systems. Also, you can safely use the rind of lemons, oranges, grapefruit, and other fruits to make zest, since their skin has not been treated with fungicides.

▼

◆ Go for the green! Thanks to popular demand, mainstream supermarkets now offer a wonderful variety of baby green and dark red lettuce and assorted leafy greens, such as romaine, mesclun, arugula, kale, spinach, chicory, and escarole. Iceberg lettuce is pretty much devoid of color, nutrition, and flavor, so when it comes to lettuce, go for the green (or red).

▼

◆ Eat raw foods for enzymes. Always include as much raw food in your diet as possible. These include enzyme-rich fresh fruits and vegetables, sprouts, nuts, seeds, grains, sea vegetables, and other organic/natural foods that have not been processed. Enzymes are critical to good health as they assist in the digestion and absorption of food. Sprouted seeds are an outstanding source of many nutrients and are also rich in enzymes. Raw food enthusiasts suggest that soaking nuts or seeds in pure water for 24 hours will activate their dormant enzymes. While I am not an advocate of most grains, once they are sprouted they become a living, highly nutritious and digestible food—great for topping salads or soups.

▼

◆ Add cooked, leftover vegetables to cold salads or omelets. Steamed broccoli, asparagus, or cauliflower, for example, are delicious when dressed with extra virgin olive oil and fresh lemon juice to taste.

▼

◆ Make friends with foods of the onion family. Add plenty of garlic, scallions, onions, chives, leeks, and shallots to your savory dishes for both their unique flavors and their outstanding health benefits—use both raw and cooked. Try adding raw garlic to your salads. As I said in Chapter 5, allicin (a potent antioxidant in garlic) is produced when garlic is finely chopped or crushed—the finer the chopping and the more intensive the crushing, the more allicin is generated and the stronger the medicinal effect.

▼

◆ Eat sprouts, tiny powerhouses of anti-inflammatory antioxidants. Enjoy them at every meal—including breakfast. Sprouts make a tasty addition to scrambled eggs and omelets—sprouted seeds, such as sunflower seeds, are a delightful topping on oatmeal or yogurt. Just about any seed, bean, or nut can be sprouted. Sprouts can be added to many dishes including salads, stir-fries, wraps, and even as a garnish for soups and stews. They provide great texture, crunch, cancer-fighting properties (especially broccoli sprouts), flavor, and very few calories overall. In addition, sprouts are a concentrated source of the living enzymes and "life force" that is lost when foods are cooked or not picked fresh from your own garden. Due to their high enzyme content, sprouts are also much easier to digest than the seeds or beans from which they came.

According to the International Sprout Growers Association (www.isga-sprouts.org), each kind of sprout has its own shape, taste, and texture. Here are some of the more common types you're likely to find at supermarkets or greengrocers:

ADZUKI BEAN: These very sweet lentil-shaped beans form fine, grasslike sprouts, with a nutty taste and texture. Add them to stir-fries or eat them raw.

ALFALFA: These threadlike white sprouts, with tiny green tops and a mild, nutty flavor, are a favorite in salads and sandwiches. They are often shipped in the containers in which they have been grown, and then are packaged in plastic bags or boxes by distributors.

CLOVER: An alfalfa sprout look-alike, most clover sprouts are produced from red clover; these tiny seeds resemble poppy seeds.

DAIKON RADISH: Often marketed as *kaiware,* these upright sprouts have silky stems, leafy tops, and a peppery-hot taste. They add tang to salads, sandwiches, and cooked dishes.

MUNG BEAN: This is the classic bean sprout most people are familiar with. These thick white sprouts are a staple in Asian dishes and are excellent in stir-fries, soups, and salads.

SUNFLOWER: These are mildly flavored, like alfalfas, but much crunchier.

EAT FIBER TO FIGHT FAT

◆ For maximum fiber, eat lots of raw fresh fruits and vegetables. Adding fiber to the diet helps regulate blood sugar levels, which is important in avoiding diabetes, metabolic disorders, and unwanted weight gain. Eat the skins of your fruits and vegetables if they are organic and unwaxed; the greatest fiber and antioxidant/anti-inflammatory properties are in the skin.

▼

◆ The recommended fiber intake per day is 25–30 grams. Do not forget to drink six to eight 8-ounce glasses of water every day–this is vitally important–especially because increased fiber can cause constipation if you don't drink enough water.

▼

◆ Fiber can help prevent gallstones and kidney stones as well as high cholesterol. Fiber-rich foods slow down the digestive process, preventing a rapid release of glucose (sugar) into the bloodstream.

▼

◆ Fiber can offer protection from certain types of cancer, such as breast cancer, ovarian cancer, and uterine cancer.

▼

◆ Fiber can help prevent heart disease. Soluble fiber, which is found in oats, for example, can exert a positive effect on cholesterol, triglycerides, and other particles in the blood that influence the development of heart disease.

EAT (THE RIGHT) FAT TO FIGHT FAT

Eat the right anti-inflammatory fats at each meal and snack because they are necessary to shed fat (and also for beautiful, youthful skin). In addition, we need healthy fats to help us absorb important nutrients and anti-inflammatory antioxidants from vegetables. According to a study published in the August 2004 issue of the *American Journal of Clinical Nutrition,* researchers compared nutrient absorption after eating salads with varying levels of fat.

Seven healthy men and women ate salads of spinach, romaine lettuce, cherry tomatoes, and carrots topped with Italian dressings containing 0, 6 (0.2 ounces), or 28 grams (almost 1 ounce) of canola oil on different occasions during a 12-week period. Hourly blood samples were taken for 11 hours after the meal and tested for nutrient absorption.

The study found that only negligible amounts of alpha- and beta-carotene and lycopene were detected in the blood after eating a salad with fat-free dressing. Significantly more of these substances, known as carotenoids, were detected in the blood after eating salads with reduced-fat dressing or full-fat dressings.

Researchers say this study shows that the minimum amount of fat required for optimal absorption of these nutrients from the salads is more than 6 grams of added fat. One tablespoon of extra virgin olive oil contains 14 grams of fat, more than enough to absorb all the nutrients in the salad. You can also drizzle a little olive oil over cooked vegetables such as broccoli or asparagus. Adding avocado slices or nuts to your salad will also give you a healthy serving of the right fats for optimum nutrition and nutrient absorption.

SLIMMING SEASONINGS AND CONDIMENTS

◆ Season your fish, poultry, vegetables, and even fruit–yes, fruit–liberally with a variety of fresh and dried herbs and spices. Try an apple sprinkled with cinnamon, a pear with a pinch of ginger, or strawberries with a splash of balsamic vinegar. Nothing in the plant world can rival the many medicinal properties of spices, from helping to lower and stabilize blood sugar, offering protection from free radical damage, providing antiaging benefits, and helping to speed up the metabolism. Cinnamon and turmeric, for example, are proven blood sugar stabilizers. A recent study found that just one-half teaspoon of cinnamon a day significantly reduces blood sugar levels in diabetics. Another study showed that in addition to its positive effect on blood sugar, curcumin, the substance that gives the spice turmeric its distinctive yellow color, stopped the changes caused by excessive alcohol consumption that lead to liver damage. In Chapter 9 you will discover many recipes that contain these herbs and spices. Note, however, that herbs and spices contain many powerful constituents. If you are taking prescription drugs, blood thinners, or have any health problem or condition, check with your physician to make sure there are no contraindications with a particular herb or spice.

▼

- Introduce a sugar-free salsa to your condiment list. To learn more about what I mean when I say "sugar-free," read the Sweeteners to Avoid sidebar later in this chapter. Salsas contain hot peppers, whose active ingredient, capsaicin, speeds up the body's metabolism. In addition, capsaicin stimulates the production of saliva, which in turn stimulates the digestive process.

▼

- DO NOT use bottled dressing on your salads—most of them contain more chemicals than your local dry cleaning plant. Instead, use fresh lemon juice and a little extra virgin olive oil to taste. The olive oil has powerful anti-inflammatory properties and is critical for absorbing the optimum anti-inflammatory antioxidants from the vegetables in the salad. Fats with anti-inflammatory action are **monounsaturated** and include extra virgin olive oil and foods rich in essential fatty acids (foods like salmon, coconut, avocados, açaí, olives, nuts, and seeds). Animal fats are inflammatory **saturated** fats, so use them in moderation. I recommend limiting your intake of red meats and full-fat dairy products. Choose low-fat dairy products and opt for fish, poultry, or tofu as a protein choice.

▼

- Keep a fresh supply of unsalted, natural nuts and seeds in your freezer. These can be added to salads and stir-fries for a wonderful crunch, delicious flavor, and those all important, slimming, essential fatty acids!

WEIGHT-LOSS WISDOM ON GRAINS, BEANS, AND LEGUMES

◆ Limit your intake of grains and beans for optimum weight loss on the 14-day plan (except for having old-fashioned oatmeal for breakfast). Instead of eating a serving of dried beans, use them to garnish salads. These foods are great sources of low-glycemic carbohydrates, as well as anti-inflammatory antioxidants and fiber, but they are more calorie-dense, so use in moderation to help accelerate weight loss. You may include more of these foods once you have reached your weight-loss goal.

▼

◆ Choose old-fashioned oatmeal as opposed to instant. By instant we mean oatmeal that is prepared by opening a packet and pouring boiling water over it. Avoid this highly processed form of a wonderful, delicious food.

▼

◆ Look for Foods Alive Organic Golden Flax Crackers at your natural food stores. These wonderful crackers have all the health benefits of omega-3-rich flaxseed; from lowering blood pressure and reducing cholesterol, to stabilizing blood sugar and relieving constipation. These flax crackers have a fresh crisp taste, and each serving provides 32 to 42 percent of the daily recommendation for fiber intake. They are also a great wheat alternative since they contain no gluten. This brand of flax crackers is not baked or fried; they are dehydrated at a very low temperature to preserve as much nutrition and enzyme activity as possible. All they contain are organic flaxseed and Bragg Liquid Aminos, a Certified NON-GMO (not a genetically modified organism aka "FrankenFood.") liquid protein concentrate, derived from soybeans. To learn more and/or to find a store near you, go to www.foodsalive.com and also visit our Resource Guide at the back of the book.

GOOD NEWS ABOUT CHOCOLATE AND COCOA

A number of scientific studies have found that both cocoa and dark chocolate with a high cocoa content contain many heart-healthy antioxidants. They contain a compound called flavonoids, which may help prevent the oxidation of LDL "bad" cholesterol and raise HDL "good" cholesterol levels in the blood. However, it is important to remember that not all chocolate is created equal when it comes to health benefits.

Cocoa butter is a heart-healthy fat that does not raise cholesterol levels. It actually contains a variety of healthy fatty acids, including stearic acid (35 percent), oleic acid (omega-9 to 35 percent), palmitic acid (25 percent), and linoleic acid (omega-6 to 3 percent). Oleic acid is also found in extra virgin olive oil and may actually raise the levels of good HDL fats in the blood.

The antioxidants in cocoa can also help improve immune function and reduce the inflammation of blood vessels. Other benefits of chocolate include:

◆ potentially lowers levels of LDL "bad" cholesterol
◆ decreases platelet "clumping" in our blood vessels
◆ regulates immune response

The darker the chocolate, the greater the cocoa content and therefore the higher the health-promoting flavonoid content, which is found in cocoa butter and cocoa solids—not in milk chocolate where the chocolate is adulterated with dairy and other ingredients.

Pure unsweetened cocoa powder is the finest way to enjoy the benefits of chocolate—without the fat and the sugar. Sprinkle it on yogurt and/or berries, use in Mexican mole sauces and, for old-fashioned hot chocolate, mix with a little milk and stevia (an herbal sugar substitute—see the following for more information).

Look for high-quality chocolates with their main ingredients being cocoa butter and cocoa solids. These include Lindt and Ecco Bello. Lindt Excellence offers an 85 percent cocoa dark chocolate bar; one serving (⅖ of a bar) has 8 grams of carbohydrate, 4 grams of protein, and 3 grams of fiber. Ecco Bello makes an organic dark chocolate bar with *cranberry seed oil* for omega-3 fatty acids, plus blueberry extract, and the powerful antioxidants *lutein, lycopene,* and *astaxanthin.*

As long as we choose the right form of chocolate and enjoy it in moderation (one to two ounces per day), there is no reason why we must give up this aptly named "food of the gods." But, remember, on a weight-loss program we may want to limit our indulgence to once or twice a week until we have achieved our desired results.

HIDDEN DANGERS IN FOODS

There are entire aisles that you should completely avoid in the traditional supermarket. These include the aisles featuring packaged cereals (other than old-fashioned oatmeal), soda and snack foods, bottled salad dressing filled with chemicals and additives, all of the aisles offering processed sugar and starchy bake mixes, puddings, cookies, juices, preprepared meals, and the rows and rows of unhealthy baked goods, filled with refined flours, chemical additives, and the deadly trans-fatty acids and unhealthy vegetable oils.

We have to take personal responsibility for our food choices. For years trans-fatty acids, which are found in foods such as vegetable shortening, some margarines, crackers, candies, cookies, snack foods, commercial peanut butter, fried foods, baked goods, salad dressings, and other processed foods have been popular food ingredients. According to an article in *Science Daily,* Dana-Farber Cancer Institute researchers have identified a molecular mechanism in the liver that explains, for the first time, how consuming foods rich in saturated fats and trans-fatty acids causes elevated blood levels of cholesterol and triglycerides and increases one's risk of heart disease and certain cancers. However, even though we now know the indisputable dangers of trans fats, and that nearly 13 million Americans suffer from coronary heart disease, and more than 500,000 die each year from causes related to coronary heart disease—they are still allowed in foods! And there is no ban in site, although the good news is that the Food and Drug Administration has now required that food labels list the amount of trans-fatty acids in food products beginning January 1, 2006.

Keep shopping simple. To be safe from possible dangers, I recommend avoiding MSG, aspartame, and food additives listed as natural flavoring, yeast extract, textured protein, soy protein extract, and so on, all of which are excitotoxins (agents that bind to a nerve cell receptor, stimulate the cell, and damage it or causes its death). Buy your foods in their most natural, unprocessed state. Learn to carefully read labels. Limit your shopping to the fresh produce, dairy, and fresh fish and poultry departments.

THE HIDDEN DANGERS OF SODIUM NITRITE

Sodium nitrite is a popular additive in hot dogs, bacon, and other cured foods such as ham and sausage. Nitrites in food can lead to formation of small amounts of powerful

Hidden Dangers of MSG

Many experts believe that monosodium glutamate (MSG) is addictive and a significant contributor to the obesity epidemic. Manufacturers of MSG even admit that it is added to foods to enhance the flavor and make people eat more! Fast-food restaurants rely heavily on MSG and we all know that fast food can be addictive.

MSG is the sodium salt of glutamate—one of the more commonly known excitotoxins. This means that in addition to potentially contributing to unwanted weight gain, MSG can kill neurons (brain cells).

According to Russell Blaylock, M.D., the following ingredients contain or may contain MSG.

Food Additives That ALWAYS Contain MSG

Monosodium glutamate	Calcium caseinate
Hydrolyzed vegetable protein	Sodium caseinate
Hydrolyzed protein	Yeast extract
Hydrolyzed plant protein	Textured protein (including TVP)
Plant protein extract	Autolyzed yeast
Hydrolyzed oat flour	Corn oil

Food Additives That FREQUENTLY Contain MSG

Malt extract	Flavoring
Malt flavoring	Natural flavors/flavoring
Bouillon	Natural beef or chicken flavoring
Broth	Stock
Seasoning	Spices

Food Additives That MAY Contain MSG or Excitotoxins

Carrageenan	Enzymes
Soy protein concentrate	Soy protein isolate
Whey protein concentrate	

cancer-causing chemicals known as nitrosamines. Studies have linked consumption of cured meat and nitrites with certain types of cancer.

To be safe, if you want to eat these foods, purchase them at the health food store. Here they should be nitrite-free—but again, read the label to be sure. Nitrite-free meats will be found in the freezer department. By keeping them frozen, we avoid the potential threat of botulism poisoning, the industry's rationale for adding these chemicals to these foods. Buy in small amounts and keep frozen until ready to use.

THE DANGERS OF HIDDEN SUGARS

Hidden sugars are everywhere. If you want to avoid sugar you need to learn how to recognize it in its many disguises.

One of the most commonly used sweeteners is high fructose corn syrup. This product is used in a great variety of products because it is significantly cheaper than cane sugar. A study published in the *American Journal of Clinical Nutrition* reported that consumption of high fructose corn syrup in beverages may play a role in the epidemic of obesity. And this is the tip of the iceberg. Many nutritionists and experts believe a host of serious health problems are arising from the use of this cheap, plentiful substance. To learn more about the pros and cons of all of the available sweeteners,

Sweeteners to Avoid

Nutritive Sweeteners

Brown sugar	High fructose corn syrup	Maple syrup
Pure cane sugar	Starch	Maltodextrin
Corn sugar	Sucrose	Molasses
Corn sweetener	Syrup	Polydextrose
Corn syrup solids	Honey	Sorbitol
Corn syrup	Invert syrup	Sorghum
Dextrose	Lactose	Turbinado sugar
Fructose	Levulose	Xylitol
Fruit juice concentrate	Maltose	
Galactose	Mannitol	

both natural and chemical, visit www.holisticmed.com/sweet/. Another site with comprehensive information on this topic is www.mercola.com.

ZSWEET™

ZSweet™ is a new, all-natural sweetener that might provide a safer alternative to chemical sugar substitutes. According to the manufacturer, it flows, looks, and tastes like sugar without an unpleasant aftertaste. ZSweet™ contains no artificial components (not even in trace amounts) and contains no caloric or sugar or carbohydrate fillers.

ZSweet™ is a patent-pending blend of Erythritol (pronounced EE-RITH-RITOL) and natural flavor enhancers. All of the ingredients in ZSweet™ are generally recognized as safe by the Food and Drug Administration and found in common fruits and vegetables. ZSweet™ does not use herbal extracts or dietary supplement ingredients and does not chemically alter any natural ingredients.

Erythritol is a new sugar substitute (sugar alcohol) similar to those familiar sugar-free ingredients such as sorbitol and xylitol. However, Erythritol enjoys significant qualities providing improved consumer benefit, including 0 calorie content, high digestibility, and consumer tolerability, and is made by natural fermentation.

ZSweet™ is the only all-natural granular sweetener that is approved for food use as a bulk consumer use product and for use in food labeled applications. The product has been developed with a sweetness profile slightly greater than table sugar (sucrose).

It can be used in the blender, over cereal, in hot or cold beverages, and is ready for baking.

The Agave Alternative

Agave nectar is made from the fruit of the agave, a cactuslike plant native to Mexico. The Blue Weber Tequilana type of agave is 25 percent sweeter than sugar and has a glycemic index of 10–11. Agave plants are in the same family as the Blue Agave, from which tequila is made. Agave nectar can be used to sweeten any type of beverage or food and may well be a healthy alternative to traditional nutritive and nonnutritive sweeteners.

Non-nutritive sweeteners (also called artificial or noncaloric sweeteners): **I do not recommend any chemical sweeteners.**

- Acesulfame K
- Acesulfame K (Sunette)—Some animal studies suggest a possible cancer-promoting effect.
- Aspartame (NutraSweet®)—Although the FDA points to more than 100 scientific experiments that purportedly document the safety of aspartame, many consumers and scientists are not convinced that long-term daily intake of aspartame is completely safe, and are concerned about the growing number of foods that contain this ingredient.
- Alitame—Like aspartame, Alitame is made from amino acids. Approval is now being sought.
- Cyclamate—Banned in the United States
- Equal®—An artificial sweetener containing aspartame, dextrose, and maltodextrin
- Saccharin
- Saccharin (Sweet'N Low®)
- Splenda—Also known as sucralose, is an artificial sweetener that is produced by

Stevia Wonder

Is there a safe alternative to conventional and chemical sweeteners? There may be—and it's called **stevia.** (Of course, if you are diabetic or have problems with your insulin levels, you need to avoid sweeteners and consult with your physician.)

Stevia is a noncaloric herb, native to Paraguay, that has been used as a sweetener and flavor enhancer for centuries. It is available as liquid and powder. Stevia cannot be legally sold as a sweet- ener due to FDA regulations; however, it may be purchased in natural foods stores and even super-markets as a dietary supplement. The website www.stevia.net is an outstanding source of infor-mation on this remarkable little plant, which enjoys great popularity in Japan. Today it is also grown and used in approximately 10 other countries out-side South America, including China, Germany, Malaysia, Israel, and South Korea.

chlorinating sugar (sucrose). This involves chemically changing the structure of the sugar molecules by substituting three chlorine atoms for three hydroxyl groups. From what I can personally discern, there have been no long-term human studies on its safety.

♦ Sucralose

THE PERRICONE WEIGHT-LOSS DIET FOOD RECOMMENDATIONS

As a basic guideline, here is a list of the recommended foods for the Perricone Weight-Loss Diet:

Recommended Foods

Omega-3 seafood

Anchovies

Halibut

Herring

Mackerel

Sablefish

Sardines

Trout

Wild Alaskan salmon—Sockeye salmon has the highest amount of omega-3 of any fish: about 2.7 grams per 100 gram portion.

Additional seafood recommendations

Bass

Clams

Cod

Crab

Flounder

Lobster

Mussels

Oysters

Scallops

Shrimp

Best poultry choices

Organic, free range chicken and turkey, Cornish hens

Turkey sausage and bacon (avoid any products with nitrates also called nitrites)

▶

Best sources of protein from dairy

Plain kefir

Plain low-fat organic yogurt

Organic eggs from free range, cage-free chickens, labeled "Omega-3"

Organic low-fat cottage cheese

Organic, unsalted nuts

Almonds

Brazil nuts

Flaxseed

Hazelnuts (filberts)

Macadamia

Organic unsalted seeds

Pecans

Pine nuts (pignoli nuts)

Pistachios

Pumpkin and squash seed

Sesame seed

Sunflower seed

Walnuts

Organic grains/legumes—use in moderation for weight loss

Barley

Buckwheat

Chickpeas

Dried beans

Lentils

Old-fashioned non-instant oatmeal or whole oats

Fruits and vegetables

Apples

Arugula

Artichokes

Asparagus

Avocado

Blueberries, blackberries, strawberries, raspberries (all berries)

Bamboo shoots

Fresh lemons

Grapefruit

Greens (turnip, collard, mustard, dark lettuce)

Green beans

Jerusalem artichoke

Kale

Green and red bell peppers

Bok choy

Broccoli

Broccoli rabe

Brussels sprouts

Cabbage

Cauliflower

Cantaloupe and honeydew melon

Celery

Cherries

Chicory

Chinese cabbage

Collards

Cucumbers

Dark green leafy lettuces (baby greens)

Eggplant

Endive

Escarole

Hot peppers

Mushrooms

Onions, garlic, chives, leeks,
    scallions, etc.

Pears

Pea pods

Radish

Rutabaga

Swiss chard

Spinach

Sprouts of all kinds

Summer squash

Tomatoes

Turnips

Water chestnut

Zucchini

Herbs and spices

Anise

Allspice

Basil

Bay leaf

Caraway

Cardamom

Cayenne

Celery seed

Chili flakes

Chives

Chervil

Cilantro

Cinnamon sticks

Ginger

Lemon balm

Mace

Marjoram

Mint

Nutmeg

Oregano

Paprika (sweet and hot)

Parsley

Peppercorns (black, green, white, pink)

Rosemary

Sage

Saffron

▶

Clove	Savory
Coriander	Tarragon
Cumin	Turmeric
Dill	Thyme
Fennel	Vanilla bean
Garlic	

Beverages

Organic green tea

Organic white tea

Organic black tea

Water (pure spring water like Fiji or Poland Spring)

Açaí (found in natural food stores)

Pomegranate juice (unsweetened)

Cocoa (made with pure cocoa powder and stevia)

Sweeteners

Stevia (available at health food stores and some markets)

Agave

Healthy fats

Organic extra virgin olive oil (look for Italian or Spanish high quality)

Flax oil

Avocado

Coconut

Olives

Nuts and seeds

Chocolate (as described in text)

FOODS THAT COME WITH WARNINGS

HIGH-GLYCEMIC FRUITS AND VEGETABLES

In other books I have recommended avoiding the fruits and vegetables that have a higher glycemic index. Watermelon, for example, is high on the glycemic index because it so delightfully sweet. Does that mean we should never eat watermelon? No, it doesn't, because watermelon has relatively few carbohydrates, and is in fact, mostly water. In addition it contains the powerful anti-inflammatory carotenoid, lycopene. We cannot make carotenoids in the body, but must obtain them from our foods. The greatest sources of lycopene in fresh fruits and vegetables are watermelon, tomato, red grapefruit, and guava.

The point is that on a weight-loss diet, I recommend choosing the fruits and vegetables that are lower on the glycemic index—we need to hedge all of our bets! But overall, I believe we can enjoy the vast majority of fresh fruits and vegetables, with the possible exception of the potato, which is rapidly converted to sugar.

Just remember to eat your protein first and save the sweet fruit or baked winter squash for the end of the meal.

Dried fruits (raisins, dates, prunes, figs, etc.) are very high in anti-inflammatory antioxidants and fiber. But they are also very calorie- and sugar-dense. When you have reached your weight-loss goal, you may add a teaspoon of chopped dried fruits to your yogurt or oatmeal.

GRAINS AND BEANS

Perricone readers know I am not a huge advocate of grains such as wheat. When you have achieved your weight goals, you may add lentils, beans, buckwheat, and barley to your diet. These foods are great sources of protein, anti-inflammatory phytochemicals, and fiber.

PRO-INFLAMMATORY FOODS TO AVOID

A simple rule of thumb is to consider the following: if it contains flour and/or sugar or other sweetener, it will be pro-inflammatory. For the most part, avoid the following foods:

Foods to Avoid

Bagels

Breads, rolls, baked goods

Cake

Candy

Cereals (except old-fashioned oatmeal)

Cheese (except, sparingly, hard cheeses such as
Romano and Parmesan, soy, feta, and cheese
made with goat or sheep's milk)

Cookies

Cornstarch

Corn bread, corn muffins

Corn syrup

Crackers (except flaxseed crackers)

Croissants

Donuts

Egg rolls

Fast food

Flour

French fries

Fried foods

Fruit juice—eat the fruit instead

Granola

Honey

Hot dogs

Ice cream, frozen yogurt, Italian ices

Jams, jellies, and preserves

Margarine

Molasses

Muffins

Noodles

Pancakes

Pasta

Pastry

Peanut butter made with hydrogenated oils

Pie

Pita bread

Pizza

Popcorn

Potatoes

Pudding

Relish

Rice

Sherbet

Shortening

Snack foods including: potato chips, pretzels,
corn chips, rice and corn cakes, etc.

Soda

Sorbets

Sugar

Tacos

Tortillas

Vegetable oils (other than olive or coconut)

Waffles

You now have a wealth of information at your fingertips about what foods to eat (and what foods not to eat), what supplements can help you attain your weight-loss goals, and how exercise and a reduced-stress lifestyle can support your overall health and well-being. It's time to put it all together. We're ready to begin the program!

Chapter 9

===

The 14-Day Perricone
Weight-Loss Diet

History will be kind to me, for I intend to write it.
— WINSTON CHURCHILL

Armed with the information contained in this book, you too can write your very own history. A solid grasp of what constitutes the anti-inflammatory lifestyle guarantees that you will be in the driver's seat when it comes to taking care of your physical and mental well-being—including the ability to maintain a healthy weight for life.

My years of research have proven beyond any doubt that the anti-inflammatory diet is the key. Inflammatory foods cause us to store fat and prevent our accessing fat for energy. They also trigger food cravings and stimulate the appetite. Anti-inflammatory foods encourage the burning of fat for energy, eliminate food cravings, and do not stimulate the appetite. Think about it. When was the last time you sat down in front of a box of cookies, bag of potato chips, or a coffee cake and had just one or two cookies, a couple of chips, or small slice of cake? More often than not, we discover that we have pretty much demolished the cookies, chips, or cake—at one sitting! And to make matters worse, we discover that we are hungry again a short time later. I think we can all agree that this is an all too common occurrence.

Now, when was the last time you did the same thing with an apple? Did you ever find that you had unwittingly eaten the entire five-pound bag? I didn't think so. How about a large green leafy salad? Did you ever find yourself eating three or four large bowls of salad—insatiable and unable to stop? Or, a grilled chicken breast or salmon fillet—were you ever able to eat three or four at one sitting and still crave more? I think most people would answer no, because these foods do not trigger the appetite in the same way that high-glycemic carbohydrates do. And they provide satiety at much fewer calories—satiety that will stay with us for many hours.

THE PERRICONE WEIGHT-LOSS DIET RECIPE FILE

My ongoing search to find the best experts, the most knowledgeable and talented people in their field, has led me to Cheryl Forberg, R.D. Cheryl is not only a registered dietitian, she is a highly successful, professional gourmet chef in that most demanding and competitive of cities, San Francisco, home to some of the finest chefs in the world. In addition, Cheryl is the consulting dietitian to the TV hit *The Biggest Loser,* a weight-loss reality show.

As a trained chef and an expert in diet and antiaging nutrition, she is uniquely qualified to develop delicious recipes that promote weight loss while they slow the aging clock.

Cheryl's book, *Stop the Clock! Cooking* attests to her excellent grasp of the antiaging power of foods. Working with our anti-inflammatory principles, Cheryl has adapted outstanding recipes from her book for the Perricone Weight-Loss Diet. We are delighted to present them here.

A special note on these wonderful recipes: spices such as turmeric, ginger, curry, and so on are antioxidant, anti-inflammatory miracle foods. The recipes reprinted here provide outstanding opportunities to sample their magic.

For the days and nights that you need a meal with minimum preparation, remember that you can always just simply grill or bake a salmon fillet, piece of fish, or chicken breast lightly drizzled with a little olive oil. Serve with a fresh lemon wedge. Also wild Alaskan salmon comes in convenient cans—great for a fast burger or addition to a salad. A quick, simple but delicious lunch or snack could be canned salmon prepared like tuna salad served on flax crackers. Add an apple and a bottle of water and you have a filling, high-fiber, nutritious yet slimming meal. Just remember, every meal should have protein, low-glycemic carbohydrates, and essential fats.

And remember that when you go out to eat, you can ask questions, then specify exactly what you want and how you want it cooked. Ask for fish or chicken that is grilled, broiled, or baked (not fried). Stay away from heavy sauces. Ask for salad with no dressing, and then sprinkle lightly with olive oil and a squeeze of fresh lemon.

A quick snack can always be two thin slices of all-natural turkey breast from the deli with a piece of fruit and a couple of nuts.

A note on portion size: I recommend a 6-ounce dinner portion of chicken or fish for women and a 6- to 8-ounce portion for men or highly active athletic women. Lunch portions should be 4 to 6 ounces for women and 6 to 8 ounces for men. While you're trying to lose weight, choose the smaller portion. Increase portion size if desired when weight loss has been achieved.

As for diet sodas, chemical sweeteners, and the like, they may not be calorie-laden, but that doesn't mean they're good for you. I recommend that you avoid man-made ingredients when possible—stick to pure and natural for best results!

THE 14-DAY PERRICONE WEIGHT-LOSS PROGRAM

Day 1.

BREAKFAST:

    2 poached omega-3 eggs with **Indian Spinach** (see recipe at end of chapter)

    2 slices turkey bacon

    ½ cup honeydew with 1 teaspoon chopped fresh mint

    8 ounces green tea with slice of ginger or spring water

        Supplements:

    1 packet of Weight Management supplements

    1 1,000 mg fish oil capsule

    1 astaxanthin capsule

    ½ teaspoon glutamine powder—mix in water and drink immediately

LUNCH:

    1½ cups **African Groundnut Stew** (see recipe at end of chapter)

    1 cup of salad (dark green leafy lettuce, dressed with 1 tablespoon extra virgin olive oil; fresh lemon juice to taste)

    ⅓ cup berries

    8 ounces spring water

Supplements:

1 packet of Weight Management supplements

1 1,000 mg fish oil capsule

1 astaxanthin capsule

½ teaspoon glutamine powder–mix in water and drink immediately

SNACK:

¼ cup **Edamame Guacamole** (see recipe at end of chapter) + 1 tsp flaxseed served with celery and jicama sticks

8 ounces spring water

DINNER:

Poached or grilled salmon (6–8 ounces raw weight) with **Spring Roll Salad** (see recipe at end of chapter)

Steamed asparagus

2-inch wedge of cantaloupe

8 ounces spring water

Supplements:

1 packet of Weight Management supplements

1 1,000 mg fish oil capsule

½ teaspoon glutamine powder–mix in water and drink immediately

BEDTIME:

¼ cup plain yogurt with ½ teaspoon vanilla

1 teaspoon ground flax

¼ cup raspberries

Moroccan Mint Tea (see recipe at end of chapter) or spring water

Day 2.

BREAKFAST:

2 soft-boiled eggs

½ cup (measured dry) **Stop the Clock! Cereal** (see recipe at end of chapter) with 1 tablespoon POM Wonderful pomegranate juice or pure açaí pulp

½ cup plain yogurt with ½ cup diced cantaloupe and 1 teaspoon chopped mint

8 ounces green tea or spring water

Supplements:

1 packet of Weight Management supplements

1 1,000 mg fish oil capsule

1 astaxanthin capsule

½ teaspoon glutamine powder—mix in water and drink immediately

LUNCH:

Icy Gazpacho with Fresh Lime (see recipe at end of chapter)

Grilled chicken breast (6 ounces raw weight boneless, skinless)

1 cup of salad (dark green leafy lettuce, dressed with 1 tablespoon extra
virgin olive oil; fresh lemon juice to taste)

½ grapefruit

8 ounces iced green tea or spring water

Supplements:

1 packet of Weight Management supplements

1 1,000 mg fish oil capsule

1 astaxanthin capsule

½ teaspoon glutamine powder—mix in water and drink immediately

SNACK:

⅓ cup cottage cheese with 1 tablespoon ground flax and ¼ cup blueberries

8 ounces spring water

DINNER:

Poached or baked halibut (or salmon) (6–8 ounces raw weight boneless) with
Curried Cabbage (see recipe at end of chapter)

1 cup of cherry tomato salad with 1 teaspoon each chopped ginger, cilantro,
extra virgin olive oil; low-sodium soy sauce and fresh lemon juice to taste

1 pear

8 ounces spring water with fresh lime

Supplements:

1 packet of Weight Management supplements

1 1,000 mg fish oil capsule

½ teaspoon glutamine powder—mix in water and drink immediately

BEDTIME:

½ cup kefir

3 almonds

6 cherries

8 ounces spring water

Day 3.

BREAKFAST:

2 whole eggs plus 2 egg whites scrambled with 1 slice turkey bacon and
  Nutty Tomato Pesto (see recipe at end of chapter)

½ grapefruit

8 ounces green tea or spring water

Supplements:

1 packet of Weight Management supplements

1 1,000 mg fish oil capsule

1 astaxanthin capsule

½ teaspoon glutamine powder–mix in water and drink immediately

LUNCH:

Salmon fillet, baked or grilled (4–6 ounces raw weight boneless) with 1 cup
  Caponata salad (see recipe at end of chapter) served on mixed baby greens

½ cup raspberries

8 ounces iced white or green tea or spring water

Supplements:

1 packet of Weight Management supplements

1 1,000 mg fish oil capsule

1 astaxanthin capsule

½ teaspoon glutamine powder–mix in water and drink immediately

SNACK:

Smoothie with ½ cup kefir, 1 teaspoon ground flax, ½ cup sliced strawberries

8 ounces spring water

DINNER:

Grilled shrimp (6 ounces raw weight)

Scalloped Tomatoes with Caramelized Onions (see recipe at end of chapter)

1 cup of salad (dark green leafy lettuce, dressed with 1 tablespoon extra virgin olive
  oil; fresh lemon juice to taste)

1 apple

8 ounces spring water

Supplements:

1 packet of Weight Management supplements

1 1,000 mg fish oil capsule

½ teaspoon glutamine powder–mix in water and drink immediately

1 ounce slice smoked salmon with 2 flax crackers

1 kiwi

8 ounces spring water

Day 4.

BREAKFAST:

1 boiled egg

½ cup **Stop the Clock! Cereal** (see recipe at end of chapter)

½ cup **Blueberry Compote** (see recipe at end of chapter) + 1 cup plain yogurt

8 ounces green or white tea or spring water

   Supplements:

1 packet of Weight Management supplements

1 1,000 mg fish oil capsule

1 astaxanthin capsule

½ teaspoon glutamine powder–mix in water and drink immediately

LUNCH:

Grilled turkey burger (4–6 ounces raw weight) served on baby spinach

¼ avocado

1 apple

8 ounces iced green tea with lemon or spring water

   Supplements:

1 packet of Weight Management supplements

1 1,000 mg fish oil capsule

1 astaxanthin capsule

½ teaspoon glutamine powder–mix in water and drink immediately

SNACK:

Cantaloupe wedge wrapped with 1 ounce slice turkey breast, drizzled
   with 1 teaspoon flax oil

8 ounces spring water

DINNER:

Grilled salmon (6–8 ounces raw weight) with **Creamy Onion Sauce with Roasted Garlic
   and Thyme** (see recipe at end of chapter)

Steamed artichoke

1 cup of salad (dark green leafy lettuce, dressed with 1 tablespoon extra
     virgin olive oil; fresh lemon juice to taste)

8 ounces spring water

Supplements:

1 packet of Weight Management supplements

1 1,000 mg fish oil capsule

½ teaspoon glutamine powder—mix in water and drink immediately

BEDTIME:

¼ cup yogurt mixed with 1 tablespoon POM Wonderful pomegranate juice
     or pure açaí pulp

2 tablespoons sliced almonds

½ kiwi, diced

8 ounces spring water

Day 5.

BREAKFAST:

2 egg omelet with 2 ounces smoked salmon, fresh dill, and cherry tomatoes

⅓ cup kefir with 2 tablespoons blackberries

8 ounces green or white tea or spring water

Supplements:

1 packet of Weight Management supplements

1 1,000 mg fish oil capsule

1 astaxanthin capsule

½ teaspoon glutamine powder—mix in water and drink immediately

LUNCH:

6 ounces **Egyptian Chicken Salad** (see recipe at end of chapter)

1 cup **Broccoli Dill Soup with Lemon and Tahini** (see recipe at end of chapter)

1 apple

8 ounces spring water

Supplements:

1 packet of Weight Management supplements

1 1,000 mg fish oil capsule

1 astaxanthin capsule

½ teaspoon glutamine powder—mix in water and drink immediately

SNACK:

½ cup yogurt with 1 tablespoon chopped hazelnuts and ¼ cup diced kiwi

8 ounces spring water

DINNER:

Grilled sablefish (or salmon) (6–8 ounces raw weight skinless)

Cucumber-Tomato Salad (see recipe at end of chapter)

Brussels Sprouts with Slivered Almonds (see recipe at end of chapter)

8 ounces spring water

Supplements:

1 packet of Weight Management supplements

1 1,000 mg fish oil capsule

½ teaspoon glutamine powder—mix in water and drink immediately

BEDTIME:

½ cup cottage cheese with 1 teaspoon ground flaxseed and ⅓ cup sliced strawberries

8 ounces spring water

Day 6.

BREAKFAST:

2 hard-boiled omega-3 eggs

½ cup (measured dry) **Stop the Clock! Cereal**

⅓ cup blueberries or blackberries plus ¼ cup plain yogurt

8 ounces green tea with lemon or spring water

Supplements:

1 packet of Weight Management supplements

1 1,000 mg fish oil capsule

1 astaxanthin capsule

½ teaspoon glutamine powder—mix in water and drink immediately

LUNCH:

Poached or baked salmon (4–6 ounces raw weight boneless)

1 cup **Persian Vegetable Soup** (see recipe at end of chapter)

1 2-inch slice honeydew

8 ounces spring water

Supplements:

1 packet of Weight Management supplements

1 1,000 mg fish oil capsule

1 astaxanthin capsule

½ teaspoon glutamine powder—mix in water and drink immediately

SNACK:

Smoothie with ½ cup kefir, 1 teaspoon flax oil, pinch cinnamon, and
    2 tablespoons raspberries

8 ounces spring water

DINNER:

Grilled Miso Salmon (or Chicken) (6–8 ounces raw weight) (see recipe at end of chapter)

Sautéed spinach (or escarole) and mushrooms

1 cup of salad (dark green leafy lettuce, dressed with 1 tablespoon extra
    virgin olive oil; fresh lemon juice to taste)

1 apple

8 ounces green tea or spring water

    Supplements:

1 packet of Weight Management supplements

1 1,000 mg fish oil capsule

½ teaspoon glutamine powder—mix in water and drink immediately

BEDTIME:

1 ounce slice smoked chicken

4 walnuts

2-inch wedge honeydew

8 ounces spring water

Day 7.

BREAKFAST:

2 ounces lox

2 flax crackers

2 soft-boiled eggs

½ grapefruit

8 ounces green tea with lemon or spring water

    Supplements:

1 packet of Weight Management supplements

1 1,000 mg fish oil capsule

1 astaxanthin capsule

½ teaspoon glutamine powder—mix in water and drink immediately

Egyptian Chicken Salad (see recipe at end of chapter)

1 apple

8 ounces spring water

Supplements:

1 packet of Weight Management supplements

1 1,000 mg fish oil capsule

1 astaxanthin capsule

½ teaspoon glutamine powder—mix in water and drink immediately

SNACK:

½ cup plain yogurt with 1 tablespoon POM Wonderful pomegranate juice
or pure açaí pulp

2 tablespoons sesame seeds

⅓ cup blueberries

8 ounces spring water

DINNER:

Pan-Roasted Salmon with Wilted Chard and Tomato-Mint Raita (see recipe at
end of chapter)

1 cup of salad (dark green leafy lettuce, dressed with 1 tablespoon extra
virgin olive oil; fresh lemon juice to taste)

1 pear

8 ounces white or green tea with lemon or spring water

Supplements:

1 packet of Weight Management supplements

1 1,000 mg fish oil capsule

½ teaspoon glutamine powder—mix in water and drink immediately

BEDTIME:

½ cup cottage cheese with 1 diced apple and 4 slivered almonds

8 ounces water

Day 8.

BREAKFAST:

½ cup cooked old-fashioned oatmeal, topped with 2 tablespoons yogurt,
¼ cup blueberries and 2 tablespoons sesame seeds

3 slices soy or turkey bacon

8 ounces green tea or spring water

   Supplements:

1 packet of Weight Management supplements

1 1,000 mg fish oil capsule

1 astaxanthin capsule

½ teaspoon glutamine powder–mix in water and drink immediately

LUNCH:

Halibut or salmon fillet, grilled, poached, or steamed (4–6 ounces raw weight boneless)

Miso Soup with Wilted Greens and Roasted Tomatoes (see recipe at end of chapter)

1 pear

8 ounces green tea or spring water

   Supplements:

1 packet of Weight Management supplements

1 1,000 mg fish oil capsule

1 astaxanthin capsule

½ teaspoon glutamine powder–mix in water and drink immediately

SNACK:

½ cup cottage cheese with 2 tablespoons salsa and 2 teaspoons sesame seeds

8 ounces spring water

DINNER:

Curried Stew with chicken, turkey, or tofu (see recipe at end of chapter)

1 cup of salad (dark green leafy lettuce, dressed with 1 tablespoon extra virgin olive oil; fresh lemon juice to taste)

½ cup mixed berries

8 ounces spring water

   Supplements:

1 packet of Weight Management supplements

1 1,000 mg fish oil capsule

½ teaspoon glutamine powder–mix in water and drink immediately

BEDTIME:

1 hard-boiled egg

Celery sticks and 2 tablespoons hummus

8 ounces spring water

Day 9.

BREAKFAST:

2 whole eggs plus 1 egg white omelet with 3 tablespoons **Baba Ghanouj**
(see recipe at end of chapter)

6 cherry tomatoes, halved, and 1 teaspoon chopped cilantro

¾ cup plain yogurt with 2 tablespoons chopped almonds and
¼ teaspoon pure vanilla extract

½ grapefruit

8 ounces white or green tea or spring water

Supplements:

1 packet of Weight Management supplements

1 1,000 mg fish oil capsule

1 astaxanthin capsule

½ teaspoon glutamine powder–mix in water and drink immediately

LUNCH:

Tomato Avocado Soup with Fresh Crab Meat (see recipe at end of chapter)

1 cup of salad (dark green leafy lettuce, dressed with 1 tablespoon extra
virgin olive oil; fresh lemon juice to taste)

½ cup black raspberries

8 ounces iced green tea with lemon or spring water

Supplements:

1 packet of Weight Management supplements

1 1,000 mg fish oil capsule

1 astaxanthin capsule

½ teaspoon glutamine powder–mix in water and drink immediately

SNACK:

Smoothie with ½ cup kefir, ¼ cup almond milk, and 6 (pitted) cherries

8 ounces spring water

DINNER:

Grilled Chicken (or salmon) (6–8 ounces raw weight boneless skinless)
with **Pomegranate Walnut Sauce** (see recipe at end of chapter)

Steamed kale

1 sliced pear

8 ounces **Moroccan Mint Tea** (see recipe at end of chapter) or spring water

Supplements:

1 packet of Weight Management supplements

1 1,000 mg fish oil capsule

½ teaspoon glutamine powder—mix in water and drink immediately

BEDTIME:

2 ounces thinly sliced turkey breast

4 almonds

2-inch wedge honeydew

8 ounces spring water

Day 10.

BREAKFAST:

3 egg omelet made with 2 egg whites, 1 whole egg, ¼ cup chopped roasted
bell pepper, 2 tablespoons sautéed red onion, and 1 teaspoon chopped basil

½ cup (measured dry) **Stop the Clock! Cereal** (see recipe at end of chapter) cooked
with water and ½ teaspoon ground cinnamon

½ cup fresh blueberries

8 ounces green tea or spring water

Supplements:

1 packet of Weight Management supplements

1 1,000 mg fish oil capsule

1 astaxanthin capsule

½ teaspoon glutamine powder—mix in water and drink immediately

LUNCH:

Asian Salad with grilled tofu or chicken breast (6 ounces)
(see recipe at end of chapter)

½ grapefruit

8 ounces iced green tea with lemon or spring water

Supplements:

1 packet of Weight Management supplements

1 1,000 mg fish oil capsule

1 astaxanthin capsule

½ teaspoon glutamine powder—mix in water and drink immediately

SNACK:

½ cup plain yogurt with 1 tablespoon sesame seeds and 1 tablespoon pure
açaí pulp or POM Wonderful pomegranate juice

8 ounces spring water

DINNER:

Three-Fish Etouffée with Baby Artichokes and Spicy Tomato Broth (see recipe at
end of chapter)

1 cup of salad (dark green leafy lettuce, dressed with 1 tablespoon extra
virgin olive oil; fresh lemon juice to taste)

1 apple

8 ounces white tea with ginger slice or spring water

Supplements:

1 packet of Weight Management supplements

1 1,000 mg fish oil capsule

½ teaspoon glutamine powder—mix in water and drink immediately

BEDTIME:

Smoothie with ½ cup kefir, 2 tablespoons blackberries, and 1 tablespoon POM
Wonderful pomegranate juice or pure açaí pulp

8 ounces spring water

Day 11.

BREAKFAST:

2 eggs scrambled with 2 ounces sliced smoked salmon and
1 teaspoon chopped chives

¼ cup (measured dry) **Stop the Clock! Cereal** with ¼ teaspoon ground ginger

½ cup sliced strawberries

8 ounces green tea or spring water

Supplements:

1 packet of Weight Management supplements

1 1,000 mg fish oil capsule

1 astaxanthin capsule

½ teaspoon glutamine powder—mix in water and drink immediately

LUNCH:

Grilled sesame tofu or chicken (6 ounces)

Tomato-Ginger Bisque (see recipe at end of chapter)

Sliced kiwi

8 ounces spring water

   Supplements:

1 packet of Weight Management supplements

1 1,000 mg fish oil capsule

1 astaxanthin capsule

½ teaspoon glutamine powder–mix in water and drink immediately

SNACK:

   ½ cup cottage cheese with 1 teaspoon flaxseed and ⅓ cup diced apple

   8 ounces spring water

DINNER:

   Salmon Chermoula (see recipe at end of chapter)

   1 cup of salad (dark green leafy lettuce, dressed with 1 tablespoon extra
       virgin olive oil; fresh lemon juice to taste)

   Steamed broccoli

   1 Asian pear

   8 ounces spring water

   Supplements:

   1 packet of Weight Management supplements

   1 1,000 mg fish oil capsule

   ½ teaspoon glutamine powder–mix in water and drink immediately

BEDTIME:

   1 ounce sliced turkey

   ¼ avocado

   8 ounces spring water

Day 12.

_____

BREAKFAST:

   Grilled salmon fillet (4 ounces raw weight boneless)

   6 cherry tomatoes

   ⅓ cup sliced strawberries

   8 ounces green tea or spring water

   Supplements:

   1 packet of Weight Management supplements

   1 1,000 mg fish oil capsule

1 astaxanthin capsule

½ teaspoon glutamine powder–mix in water and drink immediately

LUNCH:

Grilled chicken breast (6 ounces raw weight boneless skinless) or tofu veggie burger

1 cup **Watercress and Almond Salad with Roasted Onion Dressing**
    (see recipe at end of chapter)

½ cup cherries

8 ounces spring water

   Supplements:

1 packet of Weight Management supplements

1 1,000 mg fish oil capsule

1 astaxanthin capsule

½ teaspoon glutamine powder–mix in water and drink immediately

SNACK:

1 ounce sliced chicken or turkey breast

4 almonds

1 apple

8 ounces spring water

DINNER:

Salmon (or trout or mackerel) (4–6 ounces raw weight boneless) with **Baba Ghanouj**
    (see recipe at end of chapter)

Green beans sautéed with garlic and sesame oil

1 cup of salad (dark green leafy lettuce, dressed with 1 tablespoon extra
    virgin olive oil; fresh lemon juice to taste)

Sliced pear

8 ounces green or white tea or spring water

   Supplements:

1 packet of Weight Management supplements

1 1,000 mg fish oil capsule

½ teaspoon glutamine powder–mix in water and drink immediately

BEDTIME:

½ cup yogurt with 1 tablespoon POM Wonderful juice or pure açaí pulp

4 almonds

1 peach

8 ounces spring water

Day 13.

BREAKFAST:

2 egg omelet with ½ ounce feta cheese, 3 cherry tomatoes, halved,
and 1 teaspoon chopped green onion

2 links turkey sausages

½ cup blueberries

3 almonds

8 ounces spring water

Supplements:

1 packet of Weight Management supplements

1 1,000 mg fish oil capsule

1 astaxanthin capsule

½ teaspoon glutamine powder–mix in water and drink immediately

LUNCH:

Caribbean Fish Burger (see recipe at end of chapter) over baby greens

½ cup sliced tomatoes

¼ cup **Edamame Guacamole** or ¼ sliced avocado

½ cup black raspberries

8 ounces iced green or white tea or spring water

Supplements:

1 packet of Weight Management supplements

1 1,000 mg fish oil capsule

1 astaxanthin capsule

½ teaspoon glutamine powder–mix in water and drink immediately

SNACK:

1 ounce sliced turkey

2 flax crackers

2-inch slice honeydew

8 ounces spring water

DINNER:

Salmon/fish **Mole with Pumpkin and Sunflower Seeds** (see recipe at end of chapter)

Steamed artichoke

1 cup of salad (dark green leafy lettuce, dressed with 1 tablespoon extra
virgin olive oil; fresh lemon juice to taste)

1 apple

8 ounces green tea or spring water

> *Supplements:*

1 packet of Weight Management supplements

1 1,000 mg fish oil capsule

½ teaspoon glutamine powder—mix in water and drink immediately

BEDTIME:

½ cup yogurt topped with 2 teaspoons sesame seeds

1 pear

Day 14.

BREAKFAST:

2 eggs, scrambled with chopped green onion and bell pepper

1 ounce lox

½ cup (measured dry) **Stop the Clock! Cereal** with 1 teaspoon flaxseed
and 1 tablespoon sesame seeds

½ grapefruit

8 ounces green or white tea with fresh lemon or spring water

> *Supplements:*

1 packet of Weight Management supplements

1 1,000 mg fish oil capsule

1 astaxanthin capsule

½ teaspoon glutamine powder—mix in water and drink immediately

LUNCH:

Sesame Seed–Encrusted Salmon (see recipe at end of chapter)

Arugula salad with extra virgin olive oil, fresh lemon juice, 3 sliced olives, and
4 cherry tomatoes

1 pear

8 ounces spring water

> *Supplements:*

1 packet of Weight Management supplements

1 1,000 mg fish oil capsule

1 astaxanthin capsule

½ teaspoon glutamine powder—mix in water and drink immediately

SNACK:

1 ounce sliced smoked turkey

4 walnuts

1 apple

8 ounces spring water

DINNER:

Spicy Fish Stew (see recipe at end of chapter)

Wilted spinach or escarole with fresh lemon juice

1 cup of salad (dark green leafy lettuce, dressed with 1 tablespoon extra
    virgin olive oil; fresh lemon juice to taste)

½ cup berries

8 ounces spring water

Supplements:

1 packet of Weight Management supplements

1 1,000 mg fish oil capsule

½ teaspoon glutamine powder–mix in water and drink immediately

BEDTIME:

Smoothie with ½ cup kefir, 6 cherries, and 1 tablespoon POM Wonderful
    pomegranate juice or pure açaí pulp

RECITES

(e.g.: D1L = Day 1 Lunch)

African Groundnut Stew—D1L

Asian Salad—D10L

Baba Ghanouj—D9B, D12D

Blueberry Compote—D4B

Broccoli-Dill Soup with Lemon and Tahini—D5L

Brussels Sprouts with Slivered Almonds—D5D

Caponata—D3L

Caribbean Fish Burgers—D13L

Creamy Onion Sauce with Roasted Garlic and Thyme—D4D

Cucumber Tomato Salad—D5D

Curried Cabbage—D2D

Curried Stew—D8D

Edamame Guacamole—D1S, D13L

Egyptian Chicken Salad—D5L, D7L

Grilled Miso Salmon (or Chicken)—D6D

Icy Gazpacho with Fresh Lime—D2L

Indian Spinach—D1B

Miso Soup with Wilted Greens and Roasted Tomatoes—D8L

Mole with Pumpkin and Sunflower

Seeds—D13D

Moroccan Mint Tea—D1 bedtime snack, D9D

Nutty Tomato Pesto—D3B

Pan-Roasted Salmon with Wilted Chard and Tomato-Mint Raita—D7D

Persian Vegetable Soup—D6L

Pomegranate Walnut Sauce—D9D

Salmon Chermoula—D11D

Scalloped Tomatoes with Caramelized Onions—D3D

Sesame Seed–Encrusted Salmon—D14L

Spicy Fish Stew—D14D

Spring Roll Salad—D1D

Stop the Clock! Cereal—D2B, D4B, D6B, D10B, D11B

Three-Fish Etouffée with Baby Artichokes and Spicy Tomato Broth—D10D

Tomato-Avocado Soup with Fresh Crab Meat—D9L

Tomato-Ginger Bisque—D11L

Watercress and Almond Salad with Roasted Onion Dressing—D12L

African Groundnut Stew

In Africa, groundnut is the name commonly used for peanut. This version uses omega-3 rich almond butter instead of peanuts. You can substitute bite-size pieces of chicken, tofu, or fish for the soybeans.

Yield: 2 quarts; 8 (1-cup) servings

1 tablespoon extra virgin olive oil
1 medium red onion, finely chopped
1 medium green bell pepper, finely chopped
½ cup chopped celery
3 garlic cloves, minced
2 tablespoons minced, peeled fresh ginger
1 tablespoon curry powder
2 large tomatoes, peeled, seeded, and chopped,
    or 1 cup tomato sauce
1 bay leaf
4 cups fat-free, low-sodium chicken or vegetable broth
3 tablespoons creamy or crunchy natural almond butter
1½ cups cooked dried soybeans, or 1 (15-ounce) can,
    drained and rinsed, or 1½ cups cooked edamame
¼ cup chopped fresh cilantro
½ pound baby spinach leaves or other fresh greens, torn into
    bite-size pieces
Salt and pepper to taste

Nutrient Analysis— per serving
Calories 189
Prot 14g
Carb 12g
Total fat 11g
Sat fat 2g
Poly fat 3g
Mono fat 5g
Choles 0mg
Fiber 4g
Sodium 313mg
Omega-3s 28mg

1. Heat olive oil in a 4-quart saucepan or Dutch oven over medium heat. Add onion, bell pepper, and celery and sauté until soft and translucent, about 5 minutes.

2. Add garlic, ginger, and curry powder and sauté until fragrant; do not brown garlic. Add the tomatoes and bay leaf and cook, uncovered, until tomatoes are slightly reduced, about 3 minutes.

3. Add the broth and bring the mixture to a boil. Reduce heat to low and whisk in almond butter until blended. Add soybeans (or tofu or chicken or fish) and cook until heated through, about 2 minutes. Stir in cilantro and spinach. Season with salt and pepper.

Adapted from Stop the Clock! Cooking © 2003 by Cheryl Forberg, R.D., published by Avery, an imprint of Penguin Group USA, Inc.

Asian Salad

*Crispy slivers of cabbage and crunchy threads of bell pepper mingle in a tangy dressing.
The salad can serve as an Asian cole slaw side dish. As an entrée, add 6 ounces of shredded
roast chicken, poached salmon, or shrimp for each main-course serving.*

YIELD: ABOUT 2 QUARTS; 6 MAIN-COURSE SALADS

DRESSING:

1/3 cup olive oil

1/4 cup golden miso

1/4 cup rice wine vinegar

1/4 cup soft silken tofu

2 tablespoons fresh lime juice

2 tablespoons low-sodium soy sauce

2 tablespoons natural unsweetened almond butter

2 tablespoons minced green onion (green and white parts)

2 tablespoons pickled ginger

1 1/2 teaspoons dry mustard

1 1/2 teaspoons minced garlic

1 teaspoon sesame oil

SALAD:

16 ounces thinly sliced cabbage (red and green) (8 cups)

1 red bell pepper, cut into thin julienne strips

1/2 large cucumber, seeded and diced

GARNISH:

3 tablespoons chopped fresh cilantro, without stems

3 tablespoons sesame seeds, toasted

Nutrient Analysis— per serving
Calories 154
Prot 4g
Carb 12g
Total fat 11g
Sat fat 1g
Poly fat 2g
Mono fat 7g
Choles 0mg
Fiber 3g
Sodium 321mg
Omega-3s 15mg

1. **Prepare dressing:** Add all ingredients to a blender or food processor and blend until smooth. Set aside. There will be about 2 cups of dressing.

2. **Prepare salad:** Combine vegetables (and chicken, poached salmon, or shrimp) in a large mixing bowl. Add 1 cup of dressing and toss well. Garnish with cilantro and sesame seeds. Pass additional dressing separately.

Adapted from Stop the Clock! Cooking © *2003 by Cheryl Forberg, R.D., published by Avery, an imprint of Penguin Group USA, Inc.*

Baba Ghanouj (Roasted Eggplant Puree)

It's a great make-ahead hors d'oeuvre. It keeps refrigerated for several days.

YIELD: 4 CUPS; 16 (2-TABLESPOON) SERVINGS

2 large eggplants (about 1½ pounds each)

Olive oil cooking spray

⅓ cup fresh lemon juice

½ cup tahini

1 tablespoon ground cumin

1 tablespoon minced garlic

2 teaspoons white wine vinegar

1 cup fat-free plain yogurt

¼ cup finely chopped Italian parsley, without stems

Salt (optional) to taste

Nutrient Analysis— per serving

Calories 31
Prot 1g
Carb 3g
Total fat 2g
Sat fat <1g
Poly fat 1g
Mono fat 1g
Choles 0mg
Fiber 1g
Sodium 174mg
Omega-3s 2mg

1. Wash and dry the eggplant. Cut off stem end. Pierce skin with a fork to prevent eggplant from bursting during roasting. **For stovetop roasting or grilling:** Place eggplant directly on grill rack or over gas burner at medium heat. Grill for about 18 minutes, turning frequently to cook evenly. Remove from heat when eggplant has become very soft. Set roasted eggplant aside to cool.

   For oven roasting: Position rack in middle of oven and preheat oven to 350°F. Lightly coat a 15 × 10-inch baking sheet with olive oil spray. Place eggplant on prepared baking sheet and bake for about 40 minutes, turning eggplant three or four times to roast evenly. Remove from oven when eggplant becomes soft.

2. When cool enough to handle, peel and discard eggplant skin. Remove most of the seeds and cut eggplant into chunks.

3. Combine remaining ingredients except parsley and eggplant in a blender jar or the bowl of a food processor. Purée until smooth. If mixture is too thick, add hot water by tablespoons to achieve the right consistency. Add eggplant chunks and blend until smooth. Adjust seasoning with salt if necessary. Garnish with finely chopped parsley.

Adapted from Stop the Clock! Cooking © *2003 by Cheryl Forberg, R.D., published by Avery, an imprint of Penguin Group USA, Inc.*

Blueberry Compote

A hint of cloves adds depth to this vibrantly colored compote with a rich texture and full flavor.

YIELD: 2 CUPS; 4 (½-CUP) SERVINGS

2 cups fresh or frozen blueberries
3 tablespoons fresh orange juice
1 teaspoon pure vanilla extract
1 teaspoon grated orange peel
Pinch ground cloves

Nutrient Analysis— per serving
Calories 49
Prot 1g
Carb 12g
Total fat 0g
Sat fat 0g
Poly fat 0g
Mono fat 0g
Choles 0mg
Fiber 1g
Sodium 5mg
Omega-3s 0mg

1. Combine all ingredients in a 1-quart saucepan. Bring to a boil over medium heat. Cover and simmer until juices are slightly thickened, about 5 minutes. Frozen berries may take slightly longer to thicken. Remove from heat and serve.

Adapted from Stop the Clock! Cooking © *2003 by Cheryl Forberg, R.D., published by Avery, an imprint of Penguin Group USA, Inc.*

Broccoli Dill Soup with Lemon and Tahini

The rich flavors of this creamy soup disguise the fact that it's remarkably light.

Yield: 1 ½ quarts; 6 (1-cup) servings

1 tablespoon olive oil

1½ cups chopped yellow onions

1 teaspoon mustard seed

4 cups fat-free, low-sodium chicken or vegetable broth

1 tablespoon chopped fresh dill or 1 teaspoon dried dill

2 cups bite-size broccoli pieces (about 8 ounces)

¼ cup pitted, chopped ripe olives

1 tablespoon tahini

1 teaspoon grated lemon peel or minced preserved lemon peel

Salt and pepper to taste

Nutrient Analysis— per serving

Calories 88
Prot 6g
Carb 7g
Total fat 5g
Sat fat 1g
Poly fat 1g
Mono fat 3g
Choles 0mg
Fiber 2g
Sodium 322mg
Omega-3s 10mg

1. Heat olive oil in a 3-quart saucepan over medium heat. Add onions and sauté until onions are just beginning to brown, about 7 minutes.

2. Add mustard seed and sauté for about 1 minute, stirring frequently. Carefully add broth and bring mixture to a boil. Reduce heat to low and simmer for 10 minutes. Add dill and broccoli and cook until broccoli is just tender, about 4 minutes. Stir in olives, tahini, and lemon peel, and season with salt and pepper. Serve immediately.

Adapted from Stop the Clock! Cooking © 2003 by Cheryl Forberg, R.D., published by Avery, an imprint of Penguin Group USA, Inc.

Brussels Sprouts with Slivered Almonds

The nutty taste of Brussels sprouts is enhanced with a pinch of nutmeg and a hint of citrus.

YIELD: 3 CUPS; 4 (¾-CUP) SERVINGS

1 pound fresh Brussels sprouts or 1 (10-ounce) package frozen
    Brussels sprouts, thawed
2 teaspoons olive oil
Salt and pepper to taste
⅛ teaspoon ground nutmeg

GARNISH:
1 tablespoon sliced almonds, toasted
1 teaspoon grated orange peel–use organic

Nutrient Analysis— per serving
Calories 79
Prot 4g
Carb 11g
Total fat 3g
Sat fat <1g
Poly fat 1g
Mono fat 2g
Choles 0mg
Fiber 5g
Sodium 28mg
Omega-3s 14mg

1. Bring 2 quarts of salted water to a boil.
2. Remove the outer leaves from the sprouts. Trim ends of bases but leave the cores intact. Add Brussels sprouts to boiling water and cook until they are fork-tender, about 8 minutes. Drain and immediately transfer to enough cold water to cover to cool. Quarter each sprout vertically. Brussels sprouts can be prepared in advance to this point and refrigerated.
3. Heat olive oil in sauté pan over medium-high heat. Sauté Brussels sprouts until they are heated throughout, about 2 minutes. (It will take slightly longer if Brussels sprouts were cooked and refrigerated in advance.) Season with salt, pepper, and nutmeg. Garnish with almonds and orange peel.

Adapted from Stop the Clock! Cooking © *2003 by Cheryl Forberg, R.D., published by Avery, an imprint of Penguin Group USA, Inc.*

Caponata (Roasted Eggplant Salad)

This Sicilian side dish can be served as a salad or a relish, and it is perfect fare for a picnic. It tastes even better if its flavors have a chance to marry for a day or so.

YIELD: 3 CUPS; 6 (1/2-CUP) SERVINGS

Olive oil cooking spray

6 cups 1/2-inch diced unpeeled eggplant (about 1 1/2 pounds)

1/2 medium red onion (halved vertically)

1 tablespoon extra virgin olive oil

1 medium stalk celery, finely chopped

1/2 cup sliced, pitted green olives

3 tablespoons tiny nonpareil capers

1/4 cup chopped sun-dried tomatoes

1 cup tomato sauce

1/4 cup red wine vinegar or balsamic vinegar

1 tablespoon unsweetened natural cocoa powder

Salt and pepper to taste

1 tablespoon chopped fresh Italian parsley, without stems

1 tablespoon chopped fresh basil leaves

2 tablespoons pine nuts, toasted

Nutrient Analysis— per serving
Calories 106
Prot 3g
Carb 13g
Total fat 6g
Sat fat 1g
Poly fat 1g
Mono fat 3g
Choles 0mg
Fiber 2g
Sodium 428mg
Omega-3s 4mg

1. Position a rack on lower level in oven. Preheat oven to 450°F. Lightly coat a 15 × 10-inch baking sheet with olive oil spray.

2. Spread the eggplant cubes out on the baking sheet. Lightly spray the eggplant with olive oil spray. Roast in the oven for 8 minutes. Turn the cubes and roast for another 8 minutes, or until softened. Set aside to cool.

3. Slice off top and bottom ends of the onion half. Place the onion on a cutting board with the trimmed bottom end facing you, and while holding the knife at a 45° angle, make thin vertical slices.

4. Heat olive oil in a large sauté pan over medium heat. Add onion and sauté until it just begins to color, about 4 minutes. Stir in celery and cook 1 minute. Stir in the olives, capers, sun-dried tomatoes, tomato sauce, vinegar, and cocoa powder. Simmer for 5 minutes.

5. Stir in the eggplant and simmer for 10 minutes. Season with salt and pepper. Stir in herbs and pine nuts. Caponata can be served hot, cold, or at room temperature.

Adapted from Stop the Clock! Cooking © 2003 by Cheryl Forberg, R.D., published by Avery, an imprint of Penguin Group USA, Inc.

Caribbean Fish Burgers

Yield: 3 servings

18 ounces raw boneless, skinless salmon, chopped fine

½ cup minced red onion

1 egg white

2 tablespoons minced, peeled fresh ginger

1½ teaspoons minced garlic

1 teaspoon ground coriander

¾ teaspoon ground cumin

¼ cup chopped fresh cilantro, without stems

1 tablespoon fresh lime juice

1 tablespoon grated lime peel

1 tablespoon olive oil

GARNISH:

1½ cups baby salad greens

1 lime, cut into 8 wedges

Nutrient Analysis— per serving
Calories 314
Prot 35g
Carb 7g
Total fat 16g
Sat fat 2g
Poly fat 5g
Mono fat 7g
Choles 94mg
Fiber 2g
Sodium 85mg
Omega-3s 3,000mg

1. Combine all ingredients in a mixing bowl. Form into three patties. (Burgers can be prepared ahead to this point.)

2. Heat olive oil in a 1-quart sauté pan over medium heat. Add patties and cook, carefully turning once, until golden brown and cooked through, approximately 6 to 7 minutes.

3. Arrange ½ cup of greens per plate. Place hot burgers on the greens, serve immediately garnished with lime wedges.

Adapted from Stop the Clock! Cooking © 2003 by Cheryl Forberg, R.D., published by Avery, an imprint of Penguin Group USA, Inc.

Creamy Onion Sauce with Roasted Garlic and Thyme

This silky sauce is delicious with turkey, chicken, or fish.

YIELD: 3 CUPS; 12 (¼ CUP) SERVINGS

1 tablespoon olive oil

7 cloves, peeled whole garlic

2 medium yellow onions, thinly sliced (1½ pounds)

¾ teaspoon chopped fresh oregano or ½ teaspoon dried

1 tablespoon balsamic vinegar

1½ cups fat-free, low-sodium chicken or vegetable broth

Salt and pepper to taste

Chopped chives

Nutrient Analysis— per serving
Calories 43
Prot 2g
Carb 7g
Total fat 1g
Sat fat 0g
Poly fat 0g
Mono fat 1g
Choles 0mg
Fiber 1g
Sodium 51mg
Omega-3s 1mg

1. Heat oil in a heavy 4-quart saucepan over medium-low heat. Add garlic and cook, stirring frequently, until light golden brown and caramelized, about 6 minutes. Do not brown garlic beyond this or it will be bitter. Add onions and cook, stirring frequently, until onions are softened and just starting to brown, about 10 minutes. Add oregano and balsamic vinegar and sauté for 2 minutes longer. Add broth and bring to a boil. Reduce heat and simmer, uncovered, for 5 minutes.

2. Transfer sauce to a blender or a food processor and purée or process until very smooth and creamy. Return to pan and heat thoroughly but do not boil. Season with salt and pepper. Garnish with chopped chives.

Adapted from Stop the Clock! Cooking © 2003 by Cheryl Forberg, R.D., published by Avery, an imprint of Penguin Group USA, Inc.

Cucumber-Tomato Salad

4 SERVINGS

½ cup finely chopped cilantro, without stems
½ cup finely chopped fresh mint, without stems
3 medium tomatoes, seeded and diced
1 English cucumber, peeled, seeded, and diced
1 yellow bell pepper, seeded and diced
Salt and pepper to taste

**Nutrient Analysis—
per serving**

Calories 38
Prot 2g
Carb 8g
Total fat 0g
Sat fat 0g
Poly fat 0g
Mono fat 0g
Choles 0mg
Fiber 2g
Sodium 16mgs
Omega 3s 4mg

1. Combine all ingredients in a mixing bowl. Serve immediately or cover and marinate in the refrigerator for 12 hours or overnight.

Curried Cabbage

Double cooking the cabbage tones down its pungency and brightens its sweetness in this creamy curried sauce. This recipe reflects cabbage's versatility in adapting to a wide range of seasonings.

YIELD: 3 CUPS; 4 (¾-CUP) SERVINGS

½ head green cabbage (about 1½ pounds), cored and thinly sliced
2 tablespoons olive oil
2 teaspoons curry powder
2 tablespoons finely chopped yellow onion
⅓ cup fat-free, low-sodium chicken or vegetable broth
Salt and pepper to taste

Nutrient Analysis— per serving
Calories 94
Prot 2g
Carb 7g
Total fat 7g
Sat fat 1g
Poly fat 1g
Mono fat 5g
Choles 0mg
Fiber 3g
Sodium 54mg
Omega-3s 10mg

1. Cook cabbage in rapidly boiling water for 4 minutes; drain well. Set aside.
2. Heat oil in large sauté pan and whisk in curry powder to make a smooth paste. Add onion and cook for 1 minute longer. Whisk in broth and cook until it thickens slightly. Add cabbage and stir to coat well. Cook just until cabbage is tender, about 2 minutes longer. Season with salt and pepper.

Adapted from Stop the Clock! Cooking © *2003 by Cheryl Forberg, R.D., published by Avery, an imprint of Penguin Group USA, Inc.*

Curried Stew

A fragrant blend of spices punctuates this robust stew. Add an additional cup of broth and serve it as a soup. For a vegetarian version, use cubes of firm tofu or garbanzo beans, or add a pound of bite-size pieces of chicken or fish.

Yield: 2 quarts; 4 main-course servings

1 tablespoon olive oil
2 cups finely chopped red onions
2 tablespoons finely chopped, peeled fresh ginger
2 cloves garlic, minced
1 cup chopped, seeded, peeled fresh tomatoes or
    1 cup tomato sauce
1 tablespoon ground coriander
1 tablespoon ground cumin
$1/2$ teaspoon ground cardamom
$1/4$ teaspoon ground cinnamon
3 cups fat-free, low-sodium chicken or vegetable broth
$1^1/2$ pounds tofu or boneless chicken or fish fillet or
    2 cups garbanzo beans
Salt and pepper to taste
$1/4$ cup chopped fresh cilantro, without stems

Nutrient Analysis—per serving (for 4 main-course servings made with garbanzo beans)

Calories 238
Prot 13g
Carb 34g
Total fat 6g
Sat fat 1g
Poly fat 1g
Mono fat 3g
Choles 0mg
Fiber 9g
Sodium 307mg
Omega-3s 7mg

1. Heat oil in a large heavy pot over medium heat. Add onions and cook, stirring occasionally, until onions are tender but not brown, about 10 minutes.
2. Add ginger and garlic; sauté until fragrant, about 1 minute. Do not brown garlic. Add tomatoes and simmer for 5 minutes. Add spices and cook until very fragrant, about 1 minute.
3. Add broth and bring to a boil. Add tofu (or chicken or fish or beans) and simmer until cooked through, about 5 minutes. Season with salt and pepper.
4. Serve hot, sprinkled with cilantro.

Adapted from Stop the Clock! Cooking © 2003 by Cheryl Forberg, R.D., published by Avery, an imprint of Penguin Group USA, Inc.

Edamame Guacamole

YIELD: 2 CUPS; 16 (2-TABLESPOON) SERVINGS

1 cup shelled edamame (about 12 ounces unshelled)

1/2 cup unflavored soy milk

2 tablespoons chopped fresh cilantro, without stems

2 cloves garlic, minced

1 teaspoon chopped chipotle chili (optional)

1 large ripe avocado

2 teaspoons fresh lime juice

Salt and pepper to taste

GARNISH:

1 tablespoon chopped fresh cilantro, without stems

Nutrient Analysis— per serving

Calories 44
Prot 3g
Carb 3g
Total fat 3g
Sat fat 0g
Poly fat 1g
Mono fat 2g
Choles 0mg
Fiber 2g
Sodium 3mg
Omega-3s 6mg

1. Cook edamame in salted boiling water for 5 minutes. Drain and cool to room temperature.

2. Combine edamame, soy milk, cilantro, garlic, (and chile, if using) in the bowl of a food processor. Process until mixture is very smooth, about 3 minutes. Set aside.

3. Peel and seed avocado and place in a medium mixing bowl. Add lime juice and mash with a fork, leaving small chunks. Add edamame mixture and stir just to combine. Season with salt and pepper. Garnish with cilantro.

Adapted from Stop the Clock! Cooking © 2003 by Cheryl Forberg, R.D., published by Avery, an imprint of Penguin Group USA, Inc

Egyptian Chicken Salad

This is a great way to use grilled chicken breasts (or shrimp) from last night's barbecue.

YIELD: 2 MAIN-COURSE SERVINGS

DRESSING:

¹/₃ cup extra virgin olive oil

3 tablespoons lemon juice

1 teaspoon chopped garlic

1 teaspoon ground cumin

SALAD:

12 ounces cooked chicken breast, cubed or shredded (or shrimp)

1 medium cucumber, seeded and diced

1 cup cherry tomatoes, halved

¹/₂ red bell pepper, diced

¹/₄ cup finely chopped scallions

¹/₄ cup minced fresh mint leaves

¹/₄ cup chopped fresh parsley

Salt and freshly ground black pepper to taste

3 cups romaine lettuce, torn into bite-size pieces

Nutrient Analysis— per serving
Calories 375
Prot 43g
Carb 14g
Total fat 17g
Sat fat 3g
Poly fat 2g
Mono fat 11g
Choles 99mg
Fiber 6g
Sodium 138mg
Omega-3s 30mg

1. **Prepare dressing:** Combine oil, lemon juice, garlic, and cumin in small bowl.

2. **Prepare salad:** Place remaining ingredients in large bowl. Pour 3 tablespoons of dressing over and toss gently. Pass remaining dressing or reserve for another use.

Grilled Miso Salmon (or Chicken)

MARINADE:

¼ cup yellow miso

2 tablespoons mirin or rice wine vinegar

2 teaspoons tamari or soy sauce

1 tablespoon chopped garlic

1 tablespoon chopped ginger

4 (6-ounce) boneless salmon fillets or boneless skinless chicken breasts or firm tofu slices

GARNISH:

2 tablespoons chopped fresh cilantro

1 teaspoon lightly toasted sesame seeds

**Nutrient Analysis—
per serving using
6-ounce wild
salmon fillet**

Calories 325
Prot 41g
Carb 7g
Total fat 14g
Sat fat 2g
Poly fat 6g
Mono fat 4g
Choles 107mg
Fiber 1g
Sodium 802mg
Omega-3s 3,230mg

1. Combine marinade ingredients in small bowl. Pour over fish or chicken or tofu in a shallow dish. Cover, refrigerate, and marinate for 2 to 4 hours. Then grill, bake, or broil. Garnish with fresh cilantro and sesame seeds.

Icy Gazpacho with Fresh Lime

The southern region of Spain is the birthplace of this refreshing summer favorite. The sweetness of plump ripe tomatoes mingles with the fresh flavors of garden vegetables, cilantro, and a hint of balsamic vinegar.

YIELD: 1 ½ QUARTS; 4 (1 ½-CUP) SERVINGS

1 large red bell pepper

2 large tomatoes or 6 plum tomatoes (about 1 pound)

1 large cucumber, peeled, halved lengthwise, seeded

½ medium yellow onion

1 cup tomato juice

½ cup chopped fresh cilantro, without stems

¼ cup balsamic vinegar

2 tablespoons fresh lime juice

Salt and pepper to taste

Nutrient Analysis— per serving
Calories 67
Prot 2g
Carb 15g
Total fat 0g
Sat fat 0g
Poly fat 0g
Mono fat 0g
Choles 0mg
Fiber 2g
Sodium 61mg
Omega-3s 1mg

1. Roast the whole red pepper under a broiler or over a gas flame, turning occasionally, until the skin blisters and chars all over. Place in a bowl and cover with a lid, or place in a paper bag and allow it to steam to loosen the skin. Carefully peel away the skin and remove the seeds. Cut the pepper into medium dice and set aside.

2. Cut half of the tomatoes, half of the cucumber, and half of the onion into 1-inch pieces and transfer to the bowl of a food processor or a blender jar. Add the roasted bell pepper and process to a purée. Transfer mixture to a medium mixing bowl. Add tomato juice, cilantro, and vinegar. Seed the remaining tomato. Cut remaining tomato, cucumber, and onion into medium dice and add to the soup.

3. Refrigerate until chilled. Add lime juice before serving and season with salt and pepper. Serve well chilled. For a less chunky gazpacho, thin with additional tomato juice.

Adapted from Stop the Clock! Cooking © *2003 by Cheryl Forberg, R.D., published by Avery, an imprint of Penguin Group USA, Inc.*

Indian Spinach

Though this classic Indian dish is usually made with spinach, it works well with other greens such as kale.

YIELD: 2 CUPS; 4 (½-CUP) SERVINGS

2 teaspoons olive oil

1 tablespoon chopped, peeled fresh ginger

1 teaspoon ground coriander

½ teaspoon ground turmeric

½ teaspoon ground cumin

½ teaspoon garam masala or curry powder

1 pound fresh spinach leaves, washed and finely chopped, or
    1 (16-ounce) package frozen chopped spinach, thawed
    and drained

Salt to taste

Nutrient Analysis— per serving
Calories 51
Prot 3g
Carb 5g
Total fat 2g
Sat fat <1g
Poly fat <1g
Mono fat 3g
Choles 0mg
Fiber 0g
Sodium 91mg
Omega-3s 2mg

1. Heat olive oil in large sauté pan over medium heat. Add ginger and spices and cook, stirring, until mixture is fragrant and begins to bubble, about 30 seconds.

2. Add spinach and cook over medium-high heat until wilted and tender, about 2 minutes. Turn frequently to ensure even cooking. Season to taste with salt. Serve hot.

Adapted from Stop the Clock! Cooking © *2003 by Cheryl Forberg, R.D., published by Avery, an imprint of Penguin Group USA, Inc.*

Miso Soup with Wilted Greens and Roasted Tomatoes

Most Japanese people eat miso soup daily as an indispensable part of breakfast. This heartier version is an easy way to enjoy miso's rich flavors and restorative powers throughout the day.

YIELD: 6 CUPS; 4 (1½-CUP) SERVINGS

Olive oil cooking spray

3 cloves garlic, unpeeled

5 plum tomatoes (about 1 pound)

1 tablespoon olive oil

¾ cup finely chopped yellow onion

1 tablespoon peeled, finely chopped fresh ginger

4 cups fat-free, low-sodium chicken or vegetable broth

2 tablespoons sweet white miso

4 ounces firm tofu, drained and cut into ¼-inch dice

1 cup fresh spinach leaves, cut in fine chiffonade

Nutrient Analysis—per serving
Calories 139
Prot 11g
Carb 13g
Total fat 5g
Sat fat 1g
Poly fat 1g
Mono fat 3g
Choles 0mg
Fiber 3g
Sodium 718mg
Omega-3s 16mg

GARNISH:

1 green onion (white and green parts), very thinly sliced

1. Preheat oven to 450°F. Lightly coat a 15 × 10-inch baking sheet with olive oil cooking spray. Wrap garlic cloves in small piece of aluminum foil. Seal tightly. Cut tomatoes horizontally into ½-inch-thick slices and arrange in one layer on the baking sheet.

2. Place foil-wrapped garlic on the baking sheet with the tomatoes. Roast garlic and tomatoes in oven, switching position of pan halfway through roasting, about 35 minutes total, or until garlic is tender and tomatoes are lightly charred. Unwrap garlic, cool slightly, and remove skin. Add garlic and tomatoes to a food processor or blender and process until puréed. Set aside.

3. Heat olive oil in a 2-quart saucepan over medium heat. Add onion and sauté until just starting to brown, about 8 minutes. Add ginger and sauté for 1 minute. Add broth and puréed tomatoes and bring to a boil.

4. Whisk in miso until dissolved in soup. Add tofu and spinach and simmer for 1 minute. Serve warm, garnished with green onions.

Mole with Pumpkin and Sunflower Seeds

Mole *(pronounced moh-LAY)* is a magical sauce with a complex blend of spices. Most Mexican families have their own prized combination. Typically, mole is made with a fragrant blend of spices and a surprising ingredient, cocoa powder. Smoky and rich, there is a subtle undertone of chocolate, which is redefined in this riot of flavors.

YIELD: ABOUT 1 QUART; 6 (¾-CUP) SERVINGS

1½ medium red onions, cut into eighths

½ cup dry red wine

¼ cup almonds, toasted

2 tablespoons pumpkin seeds

2 tablespoons sunflower seeds, toasted

1 teaspoon coriander seeds

¼ teaspoon anise seeds

2 chipotle chilies

1 teaspoon ground cinnamon

¼ teaspoon ground cloves

2 tablespoons unsweetened natural cocoa powder

2 tablespoons olive oil

1 cup chopped, seeded, peeled fresh tomatoes

½ cup finely diced green bell pepper

1 cup tomato sauce

2 tablespoons minced garlic

2 cups fat-free, low-sodium chicken or vegetable broth

Salt and pepper to taste

Nutrient Analysis—per serving served with 6 ounce chicken breast
Calories 427
Prot 62g
Carb 11g
Total fat 13g
Sat fat 2g
Poly 3g
Mono fat 7g
Choles 143mg
Fiber 3g
Sodium 298mg
Omega-3s 14mg

GARNISH:

2 tablespoons fresh chopped cilantro, without stems

1.   Combine onions, wine, almonds, seeds, chilies, spices, cocoa powder, and 1 tablespoon of the olive oil in the bowl of a food processor; process to a smooth paste.

2.   Heat remaining 1 tablespoon of oil in a saucepan over medium-high heat. Add spice paste to pan over medium heat until bubbly and fragrant, about 5 minutes, stirring frequently. If paste is very thick, add ¼ cup water. Add tomatoes, bell pepper, tomato sauce, garlic, and 1¼ cups broth to pan. Bring to a boil. Reduce heat to low,

cover, and simmer for 10 minutes. Add enough of remaining broth to achieve a smooth sauce with the consistency of thick cream.

3. Simmer until vegetables are tender, about 5 minutes. Season with salt and pepper. Served with 6-ounce serving of grilled fish, chicken, or tofu. Garnish with cilantro.

Adapted from Stop the Clock! Cooking *© 2003 by Cheryl Forberg, R.D., published by Avery, an imprint of Penguin Group USA, Inc.*

Moroccan Mint Tea

Hot mint tea is served throughout the day in Morocco. It's also delicious iced.

YIELD: 4 CUPS; 4 (1-CUP) SERVINGS

2 tablespoons loose leaf green tea or 3 green tea bags
³/₄ cup lightly packed fresh mint leaves
1 teaspoon grated lemon peel
4 cups boiling water

Nutrient Analysis— per serving
Calories 1
Prot 0g
Carb 0g
Total fat 0g
Sat fat 0g
Poly 0g
Mono 0g
Choles 0mg
Fiber 0g
Sodium 4mg
Omega-3s 1mg

1. Place tea, mint leaves, and lemon peel in a pot or small saucepan and add the boiling water. Cover and allow it to steep for 8 minutes. Using a strainer, pour the tea into small cups or heatproof glasses.

Adapted from Stop the Clock! Cooking © 2003 by Cheryl Forberg, R.D., published by Avery, an imprint of Penguin Group USA, Inc.

Nutty Tomato Pesto

Dress up an omelet or spike a sauce with this easy recipe. Experiment with different nuts, try roasted peppers instead of tomatoes, or use arugula if basil is out of season.

YIELD: 1 ½ CUPS; 18 (1-TABLESPOON) SERVINGS

1 packed cup fresh basil leaves, without stems

2 tablespoons minced garlic

2 tablespoons chopped sun-dried tomatoes

³/₄ cup almonds, toasted

¹/₄ teaspoon salt (optional)

¹/₈ teaspoon ground pepper

¹/₂ cup extra virgin olive oil

¹/₃ cup grated Romano cheese

**Nutrient Analysis—
per serving**

Calories 97
Prot 2g
Carb 2g
Total fat 10g
Sat fat 1g
Poly 1g
Mono fat 7g
Choles 1mg
Fiber 1g
Sodium 65mg
Omega-3s 8mg

1. Place the basil, garlic, tomatoes, almonds, salt if using, and pepper in the bowl of a food processor or in a blender jar. Pulse the motor until the almonds are finely chopped. With the motor running add the oil in a stream. Pulse to blend. Stop and scrape the sides down two or three times to purée evenly. Add the cheese and process for 10 to 15 seconds. Do not overprocess; the pesto should have some texture.

2. Transfer to a bowl, cover surface with plastic wrap, and refrigerate up to 1 week.

Adapted from Stop the Clock! Cooking © 2003 by Cheryl Forberg, R.D., published by Avery, an imprint of Penguin Group USA, Inc.

Pan-Roasted Salmon with Wilted Chard and Tomato-Mint Raita

Raita is a classic yogurt-based condiment, typically served with East Indian food. The cool tang of the yogurt and fresh crunch of minced vegetables are intended to balance the spiciness of curry as in this easy yet elegant salmon dish.

YIELD: 2 SERVINGS

TOMATO-MINT RAITA:

2 plum tomatoes, peeled, seeded, and diced

1 cup seeded, diced cucumber

1 cup plain fat-free yogurt or soy yogurt, which will result
    in slightly sweeter taste

2 tablespoons minced fresh mint leaves, without stems

1/2 teaspoon ground mustard

1/2 teaspoon red pepper flakes (optional)

Pinch ground cumin

Salt and pepper to taste

PAN-ROASTED SALMON:

2 tablespoons peeled, minced fresh ginger

1 tablespoon curry powder

Salt and pepper to taste

2 (6-ounce) boneless, skinless salmon fillets

2 teaspoons olive oil

2 tablespoons chopped shallot

1/2 cup fat-free, low-sodium chicken or vegetable broth

WILTED CHARD:

1 teaspoon olive oil

1 large bunch Swiss chard, stems cut from leaves and discarded, leaves torn

2 tablespoons fat-free, low-sodium chicken or vegetable broth

Salt and pepper to taste

Nutrient Analysis— per serving
Calories 400
Prot 46g
Carb 21g
Total fat 16g
Sat fat 3g
Poly 4g
Mono 7g
Choles 79mg
Fiber 4g
Sodium 420mg
Omega-3s 2,190mg

1. **Prepare raita:** Combine tomatoes, cucumber, yogurt, mint, mustard, red pepper flakes if using, and cumin in a small bowl. Season with salt and pepper. Set aside to allow flavors to blend.

2. **Prepare salmon:** Stir together ginger and curry powder and season with salt and pepper. Pat spice mixture onto top side of each salmon piece. (Salmon can be pre-

pared up to 12 hours ahead and allowed to marinate before cooking.) Heat oil in a nonstick skillet over medium heat until hot but not smoking. Add salmon, spiced sides down, and cook, covered, for 5 minutes. Turn salmon over and cook, covered, until just cooked through, about 2 minutes. Place salmon on a dinner plate. Pour off any excess oil from pan. Add shallot to skillet and sauté for 30 seconds. Stir in broth and boil until reduced by half. Pour pan sauce over salmon. Keep warm.

3. **Prepare chard:** While salmon is cooking, heat oil in a large sauté pan over medium-high heat. Add chard and broth. Cover and cook until greens wilt, stirring occasionally, about 3 minutes. Uncover; cook until juices thicken slightly, about 2 minutes. Season with salt and pepper.

4. Place wilted greens on plate with salmon. Serve raita with each portion.

Adapted from Stop the Clock! Cooking © *2003 by Cheryl Forberg, R.D., published by Avery, an imprint of Penguin Group USA, Inc.*

Persian Vegetable Soup

This flavorful soup can be varied in unlimited ways. Loaded with fiber, a 1-cup serving is rich in protein, too. The recipe adapts well to experimenting with different beans or greens instead of spinach.

YIELD: 1 QUART; 4 (1-CUP) SERVINGS

2 tablespoons olive oil

2 medium yellow onions, finely chopped

3 cloves garlic, chopped

1 teaspoon ground turmeric

1½ cups cooked garbanzo beans or 1 (15-ounce) can,
     drained and rinsed

3 cups fat-free, low-sodium chicken or vegetable broth

8 ounces cleaned, chopped spinach or 1 (8-ounce) package frozen
     leaf spinach, thawed and chopped

¼ cup chopped fresh cilantro, without stems

2 tablespoons chopped fresh dill or 2 teaspoons dried dill

Salt and pepper to taste

Nutrient Analysis—per serving
Calories 227
Prot 12g
Carb 27g
Total fat 9g
Sat fat 1g
Poly 1g
Mono fat 5g
Choles 0mg
Fiber 8g
Sodium 363mg
Omega-3s 11mg

1. Add oil to 3-quart saucepan over medium heat. Add onions and sauté until softened and just beginning to brown, about 5 minutes. Add garlic and cook for 1 minute; do not brown garlic. Add turmeric and beans. Stir well to combine. Add broth and bring to a simmer.

2. Add spinach and bring to boil. Reduce heat to low and simmer about 3 minutes. Stir in cilantro and dill. Season with salt and pepper.

Adapted from Stop the Clock! Cooking © *2003 by Cheryl Forberg, R.D., published by Avery, an imprint of Penguin Group USA, Inc.*

Pomegranate Walnut Sauce

The ancient custom of combining meat with fruit is common in Middle Eastern food. This sauce is a lighter version used in a classic Iranian stew called koresh fesenjan. *It is delicious served with salmon or chicken. Garnish with fresh pomegranate seeds if they are in season.*

Yield: 6 servings

1 tablespoon olive oil

1 cup finely chopped yellow onion

½ teaspoon saffron or turmeric

¼ teaspoon cinnamon

¼ teaspoon nutmeg

¼ teaspoon pepper

2 cups fat-free, low-sodium chicken or vegetable broth

½ cup chopped walnuts

¼ cup pomegranate syrup (see note)

Salt and pepper to taste

Nutrient Analysis—per serving served with 6-ounce wild salmon fillet

Calories 464
Prot 44g
Carb 23g
Total fat 21g
Sat fat 3g
Poly 9g
Mono 7g
Choles 107mg
Fiber 1g
Sodium 216mgs
Omega-3s 3,720mg

GARNISH:

¼ cup chopped fresh Italian parsley, without stems

½ cup pomegranate seeds (optional)

1. **Prepare sauce:** Heat oil in large sauté pan over medium heat. Add the onion and cook until softened and light golden brown, about 8 minutes. Add the spices and cook until fragrant, about 1 minute.

2. Add 1½ cups of the broth and bring to a boil. Reduce heat to low and simmer for 5 minutes. Remove from heat.

3. Place walnuts in bowl of a food processor and process until very finely ground. Add remaining ½ cup broth and the pomegranate syrup. Process until sauce is creamy and smooth. Carefully add the hot broth and onion mixture. Purée again until smooth. Return sauce to sauté pan. Bring to a boil, reduce heat, and simmer until mixture is consistency of thick cream, about 3 minutes. Season with salt and pepper. Keep warm. Serve over grilled or poached chicken or fish. Garnish with chopped parsley and pomegranate seeds (if available).

4. **Prepare pomegranate syrup:** Place ¾ cup pomegranate juice in small saucepan and bring to a boil. Reduce heat to medium low and simmer for about 15 minutes or until juice has reduced to ¼ cup.

Adapted from Stop the Clock! Cooking © 2003 by Cheryl Forberg, R.D., published by Avery, an imprint of Penguin Group USA, Inc.

Salmon Chermoula

Chermoula is a fragrant and spicy sauce commonly found in Moroccan food stalls and served with fried fish. The sauce is delicious with poached salmon, too.

<small>YIELD: 2 SERVINGS</small>

¹/₂ teaspoon ground coriander

¹/₄ teaspoon ground pepper

¹/₄ teaspoon ground cumin

¹/₄ teaspoon crumbled saffron threads (optional)

3 teaspoons olive oil

1 cup finely chopped red onion

2 tablespoons minced preserved lemon peel or 2 tablespoons
   grated lemon peel

2 (6-ounce) boneless, skinless salmon fillets

¹/₄ cup white wine

2 tablespoons chopped fresh cilantro, without stems

Salt and pepper

Nutrient Analysis— per serving
Calories 391
Prot 40g
Carb 11g
Total fat 19g
Sat fat 3g
Poly fat 6g
Mono fat 9g
Choles 105mg
Fiber 2g
Sodium 90mgs
Omega-3s 3,420mg

1. Mix spices in a small bowl. Set aside. Heat 2 teaspoons of the olive oil in a medium sauté pan over medium-high heat. Add onion and sauté until soft and translucent, about 4 minutes. Add spice mixture and sauté until richly fragrant, about 1 minute. Remove from heat and stir in lemon peel. Transfer to a small mixing bowl and set aside.

2. Return same pan to medium-high heat. Add remaining 1 teaspoon olive oil and heat until hot but not smoking.

3. Add salmon and cook for about 4 minutes. Turn salmon over and cook until just opaque, about 2 minutes. Transfer salmon to a dinner plate. Pour off any excess oil from pan. Stir in white wine and boil until reduced by half. Stir in onion mixture and simmer until heated through. Stir in chopped cilantro and season with salt and pepper.

4. Top salmon fillets with chermoula sauce and serve.

Adapted from Stop the Clock! Cooking © 2003 by Cheryl Forberg, R.D., published by Avery, an imprint of Penguin Group USA, Inc.

Scalloped Tomatoes with Caramelized Onions

Silky and sweet, caramelized onions add a rustic touch to unadorned tomatoes. Serve with roast chicken and a green vegetable. This is a great dish for a potluck, as it can be assembled a day ahead of time and baked just before serving.

YIELD: 1 ½ QUARTS; 8 (¾-CUP) SERVINGS

CARAMELIZED ONIONS:

1 tablespoon olive oil

2 large onions, halved lengthwise and cut crosswise into ⅛-inch-thick slices

¼ teaspoon salt

⅛ teaspoon ground pepper

⅓ cup fat-free, low-sodium chicken or vegetable broth

2 tablespoons balsamic vinegar

SAUCE:

¼ cup olive oil

¼ cup minced onion

2 cups fat-free, low-sodium chicken or vegetable broth

1 teaspoon Italian seasoning (mixed dry herbs such as oregano, thyme, and basil)

Salt and pepper to taste

2 pounds plum tomatoes (10 to 12 tomatoes)

Salt and pepper to taste

⅓ cup coarsely grated Parmigiana Reggiano cheese

Nutrient Analysis— per serving
Calories 140
Prot 5g
Carb 10g
Total fat 10g
Sat fat 2g
Poly fat 1g
Mono fat 7g
Choles 3mg
Fiber 2g
Sodium 272mg
Omega-3s 8mg

1. Preheat oven to 375°F. Lightly coat a 2-quart soufflé or baking dish with olive oil cooking spray.

2. **Prepare onions:** Heat oil in a large skillet over medium-high heat. Add onions, salt, and pepper; cook, stirring frequently, until onions begin to brown, about 12 minutes. Add broth and vinegar. Reduce heat to medium; simmer, stirring occasionally, until juices are nearly dry, about 12 minutes.

3. **Prepare sauce:** Heat olive oil in a heavy saucepan over medium-low heat and add onion. Simmer for about 3 minutes until onions are soft and translucent. Add broth in a stream, continuing to whisk. Bring sauce to a boil, reduce heat, and simmer until slightly thickened, about 2 minutes. Remove pan from heat and stir in seasoning and salt and pepper. Set aside.

4. Core tomatoes and cut horizontally into about ¼-inch-thick slices. Season with salt and pepper.

5. In prepared baking dish, layer one-third of tomatoes, one-third of onions, and one-third of sauce. Repeat layers two more times. Sprinkle cheese on top and bake, uncovered, for 35 minutes, or until top is golden. Serve warm.

Adapted from Stop the Clock! Cooking © 2003 by Cheryl Forberg, R.D., published by Avery, an imprint of Penguin Group USA, Inc.

Sesame Seed–Encrusted Salmon

4 (6-ounce) salmon fillets
Salt and pepper to taste
4 tablespoons white sesame seeds
2 tablespoons olive oil

GARNISH:
Fresh cilantro
Sushi ginger
Low-sodium soy sauce

Nutrient Analysis— per serving
Calories 361
Prot 39g
Carb 1g
Total fat 21g
Sat fat 3g
Poly fat 7g
Mono fat 10g
Choles 107mg
Fiber 1g
Sodium 85mg
Omega-3s 3,430mg

1. Preheat the oven to 350°F.
2. Season salmon with salt and pepper. Place sesame seeds in shallow baking dish. Brush salmon fillets lightly with oil and dredge the flesh side (not skin side) in the seeds. Heat oil in a large skillet over medium-high heat. Sear the salmon seed-side down in the pan just until it is light golden—do not burn the seeds or they will be bitter. Lightly brown skin side also. Transfer fillets, sesame seed side up, to a baking dish and place the salmon in the oven. Roast for 7 to 8 minutes. Serve the roast salmon immediately with cilantro, sushi ginger, and low-sodium soy sauce.

Spicy Fish Stew

The flavors of this stew will vary depending on the fish you select. Whatever you choose, the intriguing blend of flavors results in a dish that is elegant in its simplicity.

Yield: 1 ½ quarts; 3 servings

1 tablespoon olive oil

1 cup finely chopped yellow onion

1 cup finely chopped green bell pepper

1 cup diced, peeled, seeded tomatoes

1 ½ teaspoons ground coriander

½ teaspoon ground cumin

4 cups fat-free chicken, fish, or vegetable broth

18 ounces boneless, skinless fish fillets (salmon, tuna, or mackerel), cut into ¾-pieces

2 tablespoons tahini

1 tablespoon finely chopped preserved lemon peel or grated lemon peel

¼ cup finely chopped fresh cilantro, without stems

Nutrient Analysis— per serving	
Calories 471	
Prot 50g	
Carb 16g	
Total fat 23g	
Sat fat 3g	
Poly fat 8g	
Mono fat 9g	
Choles 107mg	
Fiber 4g	
Sodium 618mg	
Omega-3s 3,440mg	

1. Heat olive oil in a 3-quart saucepan over medium heat. Add onion and bell pepper and sauté until soft but not browned, about 5 minutes. Add tomatoes and sauté for 3 minutes. Stir in spices and simmer for 1 minute.

2. Carefully pour in broth and bring mixture to a boil. Add fish. When mixture returns to a boil, reduce heat to low. Simmer until fish is cooked through, 3 minutes.

3. Stir in tahini, lemon peel, and chopped cilantro. Serve hot.

Adapted from Stop the Clock! Cooking © *2003 by Cheryl Forberg, R.D., published by Avery, an imprint of Penguin Group USA, Inc.*

Spring Roll Salad

YIELD: ABOUT 2 (1-CUP) SERVINGS

1 tablespoon olive oil

1 medium yellow onion, finely chopped

2 tablespoons minced garlic

2 tablespoons chopped, peeled fresh ginger

3 cups finely shredded green cabbage

¼ cup chopped fresh cilantro, without stems

1 tablespoon low-sodium soy sauce

Salt to taste

GARNISH:

Cilantro sprigs

Nutrient Analysis— per serving
Calories 128
Prot 3g
Carb 15g
Total fat 7g
Sat fat 1g
Poly fat 1g
Mono fat 5g
Choles 0mg
Fiber 3g
Sodium 290mg
Omega-3s 10mg

1. Heat olive oil in a large sauté pan over medium-high heat. Add onion and sauté until softened, but not colored, 2 minutes. Add garlic and ginger and sauté for 1 minute longer. Add cabbage and stir-fry until cabbage is softened, about 2 minutes.

2. Remove pan from heat. Add cilantro and soy sauce. Stir until combined. Season with salt if desired.

Adapted from Stop the Clock! Cooking © 2003 by Cheryl Forberg, R.D., published by Avery, an imprint of Penguin Group USA, Inc.

Stop the Clock! Cereal

YIELD: 6 CUPS DRY; 12 SERVINGS

³/₄ cup water

4 cups old-fashioned oats

1 cup oat bran

¹/₂ cup nonfat dry milk

¹/₂ cup low-fat soy flour

¹/₂ cup almond meal

¹/₂ cup ground flaxseed

¹/₄ cup sesame seed

Nutrient Analysis—per serving (prepared with water)
Calories 216
Prot 10g
Carb 25g
Total fat 9g
Sat fat 1g
Poly fat 3g
Mono fat 2g
Choles 1mg
Fiber 6g
Sodium 31mg
Omega-3s 1,020mg

1. Combine all ingredients and store in freezer in airtight container.

2. **To prepare one serving:** In a small saucepan, bring water to a boil. Stir in ¹/₂ cup cereal mix and turn heat to low. Simmer for 1 minute, cover, and remove from heat. Allow to stand for 3 minutes. Serve immediately with fresh berries, if desired. (If you're in a hurry, combine cereal and water in a deep bowl and microwave for 3 minutes.)

Recipe adapted from Stop the Clock! Cooking © *2003 by Cheryl Forberg, R.D., published by Avery, an imprint of Penguin Group USA, Inc.*

Three-Fish Etouffée with Baby Artichokes and Spicy Tomato Broth

Etouffée is a spicy Cajun stew traditionally made with crawfish and vegetables.

YIELD: 2¾ QUARTS; 4 SERVINGS

¼ cup olive oil

1 cup chopped yellow onion

⅓ cup chopped red bell pepper

¼ cup ½-inch diced celery

2 tablespoons minced garlic

1 cup chopped tomatoes or 1 cup tomato sauce

2 teaspoons finely chopped fresh oregano or ½ teaspoon
    dried oregano

1 teaspoon red pepper flakes (optional)

1 cup red wine or water

4 cups fat-free, low-sodium fish, chicken, or vegetable broth

9 ounces fresh artichoke hearts, quartered or 1 (9-ounce) package
    frozen artichoke hearts, thawed and cut in quarters lengthwise

1 small bay leaf

2 ounces fresh shiitake mushrooms, stemmed, caps sliced (about 1 cup)

24 ounces (1½ pounds) assorted boneless fish fillets (such as salmon,
    mackerel, tuna), cut into 1-inch cubes

¼ cup chopped fresh parsley, without stems

1½ tablespoons finely grated lemon peel

Salt and pepper to taste

Nutrient Analysis— per serving
Calories 675
Prot 50g
Carb 57g
Total fat 25g
Sat fat 4g
Poly fat 5g
Mono fat 14g
Choles 77mg
Fiber 12g
Sodium 537mg
Omega-3s 2,240mg

1. Heat oil in a 4-quart large pot or Dutch oven over medium heat. Add onion, bell pepper, and celery and cook until tender. Add garlic, tomatoes, oregano, and red pepper flakes if using; simmer 1 minute longer. Add wine or water and bring to a boil. Reduce heat and simmer until the liquid has reduced by half, about 5 minutes.

2. Stir in broth and bring to a boil. Reduce heat. Add artichoke hearts, bay leaf, and mushrooms and simmer for 2 minutes. Add fish; cook, stirring gently, until just opaque, about 4 minutes. Stir in parsley and lemon peel. Season with salt and pepper. Serve hot.

Adapted from Stop the Clock! Cooking © 2003 by Cheryl Forberg, R.D., published by Avery, an imprint of Penguin Group USA, Inc.

Tomato-Avocado Soup with Fresh Crab Meat

YIELD: 6 SERVINGS

4 cups tomato juice

2 tablespoons finely chopped celery

1 tablespoon finely chopped onion

3 tablespoons fresh lime juice

2 tablespoons Worcestershire sauce

2 tablespoons Dijon mustard

2 tablespoons tahini

Salt and pepper to taste

GARNISH:

1½ ripe medium avocados

¼ cup fresh lime juice

¼ cup chopped fresh cilantro, without stems

24 ounces lump crabmeat (or lobster meat)

Lime wedges

Fresh cilantro

Nutrient Analysis— per serving with 4 ounces crab meat
Calories 258
Prot 28g
Carb 14g
Total fat 12g
Sat fat 2g
Poly fat 2g
Mono fat 6g
Choles 80mg
Fiber 4g
Sodium 582mg
Omega-3s 2,090mg

1. **Prepare soup:** Combine tomato juice, celery, onion, lime juice, Worcestershire sauce, mustard, and tahini in a blender or food processor. Puree until smooth. Season with salt and pepper. Cover and refrigerate until chilled or up to a day in advance.

2. Just before serving, peel and pit the avocados; cut in ½-inch cubes. Toss avocado cubes with the lime juice. Divide the avocado among 6 chilled serving bowls. Arrange 4–6 large shrimp or 4–6 ounces lump crabmeat or lobster meat with the avocados. Ladle 1 cup of soup into each bowl. Garnish with fresh lime wedges and fresh cilantro.

Adapted from Stop the Clock! Cooking *© 2003 by Cheryl Forberg, R.D., published by Avery, an imprint of Penguin Group USA, Inc.*

Tomato-Ginger Bisque

America's all-time favorite soup is spiced with ginger to give it an exotic flair. A steaming bowl served with crusty bread provides the ultimate meal of simple comfort food. Ginger is also an excellent digestive aid. If you are endowed with an abundant tomato harvest, make batches of this recipe and freeze to enjoy later.

YIELD: 1 QUART; 4 (1-CUP) SERVINGS

1 tablespoon olive oil

2 tablespoons minced shallot

4 quarter-size slices peeled fresh ginger

2 cloves garlic, peeled

4 medium tomatoes (about 1 pound), peeled, seeded,
    and coarsely chopped

1¼ cup fat-free, low-sodium chicken or vegetable broth

½ cup unflavored soy milk

Salt and pepper to taste

Nutrient Analysis— per serving
Calories 95
Prot 5g
Carb 11g
Total fat 4g
Sat fat <1g
Poly fat 1g
Mono fat 3g
Choles 0mg
Fiber 2g
Sodium 134mg
Omega-3s 8mg

GARNISH:

¼ cup fresh basil leaves, cut in a chiffonade

1. Heat olive oil in a 2-quart saucepan over medium heat. Add shallot and ginger and sauté until softened, about 1 minute.

2. Add garlic and tomatoes to the saucepan. Simmer until mixture begins to thicken, about 4 minutes. Remove slices of ginger. Add broth and bring to a boil.

3. Carefully transfer soup to the bowl of a food processor or a blender jar. Process until smooth. Return to the saucepan. Add soy milk and simmer just until heated. Do not boil or soy milk will curdle. Season to taste with salt and pepper and garnish with basil.

Note: The chiffonade cut is done by rolling the leaves lengthwise and slicing crosswise into thin slivers.

Adapted from Stop the Clock! Cooking © 2003 by Cheryl Forberg, R.D., published by Avery, an imprint of Penguin Group USA, Inc.

Watercress and Almond Salad with Roasted Onion Dressing

Peppery watercress is a welcome change from lettuce in this salad of many textures and flavors. Try it with different nuts or sprinkle with fresh berries. Extra dressing keeps well in the refrigerator for up to 1 week.

YIELD: 4 SERVINGS

DRESSING:

1 medium red onion (about 8 ounces)

¼ cup plus 1 teaspoon olive oil

¼ cup fresh lime juice

1 tablespoon Dijon mustard

3 tablespoons balsamic vinegar

Salt and pepper to taste

SALAD:

1 medium red apple

1 teaspoon fresh lime juice

4 cup watercress, washed and dried

⅓ cup chopped almonds, toasted

Nutrient Analysis—per serving
Calories 105
Prot 3g
Carb 7g
Total fat 8g
Sat fat 1g
Poly fat 4g
Mono fat 3g
Choles 0mg
Fiber 2g
Sodium 33mg
Omega-3s 34mg

1. **Prepare dressing:** Preheat oven to 400°F. Peel onion and cut into 8 wedges. Place onion, cut side down, on baking sheet. Drizzle with 1 teaspoon of the olive oil. Bake for 15 minutes. Turn onion over and bake until brown and caramelized, about 15 minutes longer. Set aside to cool.

2. Place onion in bowl of a food processor; add lime juice, mustard, and vinegar. Purée until smooth and thick. (Add 1 tablespoon of water if mixture is too thick to process.) Add the remaining ¼ cup of olive oil in a thin stream. Season with salt and pepper. Set aside. There will be about 1¼ cups of dressing.

3. **Prepare salad:** Cut apple in half vertically and remove core. Cut halves crosswise into ¼-inch-thick slices. Stack the slices and cut crosswise into ⅛-inch-wide slices, forming thin matchsticks. Toss apple sticks in lime juice in a large mixing bowl. Set aside.

4. Add watercress and nuts to the apple. Add enough dressing to coat greens, about 3 tablespoons; toss well. Divide salad evenly among 8 plates. Serve immediately. Pass extra dressing separately.

Adapted from Stop the Clock! Cooking © 2003 by Cheryl Forberg, R.D., published by Avery, an imprint of Penguin Group USA, Inc.

Appendix A

The Pros and Cons of Soy Foods

As with so many topics today, soy foods have their champions and their opponents. There appears to be comprehensive scientific research on the potential dangers of soy products, particularly unfermented soy. One potential danger is phytic acid, an acid that occurs in soy and cereal grains that when ingested interferes with the intestinal absorption of various minerals including calcium, magnesium, copper, iron, and zinc. Apparently, only fermented soy products are free of phytic acid. In addition, fermented soy increases the availability of isoflavones (one of a family of phytoestrogens found chiefly in soybeans that is under investigation for its preventive health benefits as a nutritional supplement).

The fermentation also creates probiotics—the "good" bacteria that is so critical for optimum health of the digestive tract. Probiotics are also what give yogurt and kefir their powerful health-promoting abilities. Interestingly, "pro-biotic" means "pro-life"; "anti-biotic" means "anti-life." When possible choose the life-giving options.

Fermented soy products include

♦ natto
♦ miso
♦ tempeh

- soy sauces
- fermented tofu and soy milk (which are clearly labeled as such)

The following is an alphabetical list of soy foods courtesy of the U.S. Soyfoods Directory, www.soyfoods.com (as with all other foods, avoid those with chemical additives).

Green Soybeans (Edamame): These large soybeans are harvested when the beans are still green and sweet-tasting and can be served as a snack or a main vegetable dish, after boiling in slightly salted water for 15 to 20 minutes. They are high in protein and fiber and contain no cholesterol. Edamame is more often found in Asian and natural food stores, shelled or still in the pod.

Hydrolyzed Vegetable Protein (HVP): Hydrolyzed vegetable protein is a protein obtained from any vegetable, including soybeans. The protein is broken down into amino acids by a chemical process called acid hydrolysis. HVP is a flavor enhancer that can be used in soups, broths, sauces, gravies, flavoring and spice blends, canned and frozen vegetables, meats, and poultry. Caution, may contain MSG.

Lecithin: Extracted from soybean oil, lecithin is used in food manufacturing as an emulsifier in products high in fats and oils. It also promotes stabilization, antioxidation, crystallization, and spattering control. Powdered lecithins can be found in natural and health food stores.

Meat Alternatives (Meat Analogs): Meat alternatives made from soybeans contain soy protein or tofu and other ingredients mixed together to simulate various kinds of meat. These meat alternatives are sold as frozen, canned, or dried foods. Usually, they can be used the same way as the foods they replace. With so many different meat alternatives available to consumers, the nutritional value of these foods varies considerably. Generally, they are lower in fat, but read the label to be certain. Meat alternatives made from soybeans are excellent sources of protein, iron, and B vitamins. Read ingredient lists carefully to avoid unwanted ingredients, preservatives, sugars, MSG, and so on.

Miso: Miso is a rich, salty condiment that characterizes the essence of Japanese cooking. A smooth paste, miso is made from soybeans and a grain such as rice, plus salt and a mold culture, and then aged in cedar vats for one to three years. Miso should be refrigerated. Use miso to flavor soups, sauces, dressings, marinades, and pâtés.

Natto: Natto is made of fermented, cooked whole soybeans. Because the fermentation process breaks down the beans' complex proteins, natto is more easily digested than whole soybeans. It has a sticky, viscous coating with a cheesy texture. In Asian countries natto traditionally is served as a topping for rice, in miso soups, and is used with vegetables. Natto can be found in Asian and natural food stores.

Soy Cheese: Soy cheese is made from soy milk. Its creamy texture makes it an easy substitute for sour cream or cream cheese and can be found in variety of flavors in natural foods stores.

Soy Fiber (Okara, Soy Bran, Soy Isolate Fiber): There are three basic types of soy fiber: Okara, soy bran, and soy isolate fiber. All of these products are high-quality, inexpensive sources of dietary fiber.

- Okara is a pulp fiber by-product of soy milk. It has less protein than whole soybeans, but the protein remaining is of high quality.

- Soy bran is made from hulls (the outer covering of the soybean), which are removed during the initial processing. The hulls contain a fibrous material that can be extracted and then refined for use as a food ingredient.

- Soy isolate fiber, also known as structured protein fiber (SPF), is soy protein isolate in a fibrous form.

Soy Flour: Soy flour is made from roasted soybeans ground into a fine powder. There are three kinds of soy flour available:

- Natural or full-fat, which contains the natural oils found in the soybean
- Defatted, which has the oils removed during processing
- Lecithinated, which has had lecithin added to it

All soy flour gives a protein boost to recipes. However, defatted soy flour is an even more concentrated source of protein than full-fat soy flour. Although used mainly by the food industry, soy flour can be found in natural food stores and some supermarkets. Soy flour is gluten-free.

Soy Grits: Soy grits are similar to soy flour except that the soybeans have been toasted and cracked into coarse pieces, rather than the fine powder of soy flour. Soy grits can be used as a substitute for flour in some recipes.

Soy Protein Concentrate: Soy protein concentrate comes from defatted soy flakes. It contains about 70 percent protein, while retaining most of the bean's dietary fiber.

Soy Protein Isolates (Isolated Soy Protein): When protein is removed from defatted flakes the result is soy protein isolates, the most highly refined soy protein. Containing 92 percent protein, soy protein isolates possess the greatest amount of protein of all soy products.

Soy Protein, Textured: Textured soy protein (TSP) usually refers to products made from textured soy flour, although the term can also be applied to textured soy protein concentrates and spun soy fiber. Textured soy flour (TSF) is made by running defatted soy flour through an extrusion cooker, which allows for many different forms and sizes. When hydrated it has a chewy texture. It is widely used as a meat extender. One of the more popular brands of TSF is made by Archer Daniels Midland Company, which owns the right to the product named Textured Vegetable Protein (TVP). Read ingredients carefully to ensure no MSG or other undesirable ingredients are added.

Soy Sauce (Tamari, Shoyu, Teriyaki): Soy sauce is a dark brown liquid made from soybeans that have undergone a fermenting process. Soy sauces have a salty taste, but are lower in sodium than traditional table salt. Specific types of soy sauce are: shoyu, tamari, and teriyaki. Shoyu is a blend of soybeans and wheat. Tamari is made only from soybeans and is a by-product of making miso. Teriyaki sauce can be thicker than other types of soy sauce and includes other ingredients such as sugar, vinegar, and spices. Always buy organic, naturally fermented soy, with no extra additives.

Soy Yogurt: Soy yogurt is made from soy milk. Its creamy texture makes it an easy substitute for sour cream or cream cheese. Look for plain soy yogurt in natural food stores and some grocery stores.

Soybeans, Whole: As soybeans mature in the pod they ripen into a hard, dry bean. Most soybeans are yellow. However, there are brown and black varieties. Whole soybeans (an excellent source of protein and dietary fiber) can be cooked and used in sauces, stews, and soups. Whole soybeans that have been soaked can be roasted for snacks and can be purchased in natural food stores and some supermarkets. When grown without agricultural chemicals, they are referred to as organically grown soybeans.

Soymilk, Soy Beverages: Soybeans, soaked, ground fine, and strained, produce a fluid called soybean milk, which is a substitute for cow's milk. Plain, unfortified soy milk is a source of high-quality protein and B-vitamins. Soymilk is most commonly found in aseptic containers (nonrefrigerated, shelf stable), but also can be found in quart and half gallon containers in the dairy case at the supermarket. Soymilk is also sold as a powder, which must be mixed with water.

Soy Nut Butter: Made from roasted, whole soy nuts, which are then crushed and blended with soy oil and other ingredients, soy nut butter has a slightly nutty taste, significantly less fat than peanut butter, and provides many other nutritional benefits as well. Soy nut butter can be found in a few supermarkets or through mail-order companies.

Soy Nuts: Roasted soy nuts are whole soybeans that have been soaked in water and then baked until browned. Soy nuts can be found in a variety of flavors. High in protein and isoflavones, soy nuts are similar in texture and flavor to peanuts. You can find roasted soy nuts in natural food stores and through mail-order catalogs.

Soy Oil and Products: Soy oil is the natural oil extracted from whole soybeans. It is the most widely used oil in the United States, accounting for more than 75 percent of our total vegetable fats and oils intake. Oil sold in the grocery store under the generic name "vegetable oil" is usually 100 percent soy oil or a blend of soy oil and other oils. Soy oil is cholesterol-free and high in polyunsaturated fat. Soy oil is rich in the omega-6 essential fatty acids. As my readers know, our diets contain far too many omega-6s and not enough omega-3s, so I recommend avoiding soy and other vegetable oils other than olive or flax oil.

Soy Sprouts: Although not as popular as mung bean sprouts or alfalfa sprouts, soy sprouts (also called soybean sprouts) contain protein and vitamin C. They can be sprouted in the same manner as other beans and seeds. Soy sprouts must be cooked quickly at low heat so they don't get mushy. They can also be used raw in salads or soups, or in stir-fried, sautéed, or baked dishes.

Tempeh: Tempeh, a traditional Indonesian food, is a chunky, tender soybean cake. Tempeh can be marinated and grilled and added to soups, casseroles, or chili. Found in Asian food stores.

Tofu and Tofu Products: Tofu, also known as soybean curd, is a soft cheeselike food made by curdling fresh hot soymilk with a coagulant. Tofu is a bland product that easily absorbs the flavors of other ingredients with which it is cooked. Tofu is rich in protein, B vitamins, and low in sodium.

Whipped Toppings, Soy-Based: Soy-based whipped toppings are similar to other nondairy whipped toppings, except that hydrogenated soy oil is used instead of other vegetable oils. As we have learned, hydrogenated products contain dangerous trans-fatty acids.

Yuba: Yuba is made by lifting and drying the thin layer formed on the surface of cooling hot soy milk. It has a high protein content and is commonly sold fresh, half-dried and dried. In the United States, dried yuba sheets (called dried bean curd, bean curd sheets, or bean curd skin) and U-shaped rolls (called bamboo yuba or bean curd sticks) can be found in Asian food stores.

Appendix B

Seafood Safety

Many people are worried about the safety of seafood—and rightly so. There are some forms of seafood that are safe to eat and others that we should avoid. Perricone readers know that I am a huge advocate of salmon, as long as it's wild Alaskan or Pacific salmon (see Chapter 5). Unlike farmed salmon, Alaskan sockeye salmon and all other wild Alaskan species grow free of antibiotics, pesticides, synthetic coloring agents, growth hormones, and GMOs (genetically modified organisms).

The FDA is conservative in protecting the health of American consumers. As such, it has set consumption advice for mercury at the 1 ppm (parts per million) level, which is the limit allowed by the FDA for fish intended for human consumption. The level is purposely set 10 times lower than the lowest level associated with health problems (specifically mercury poisoning). This conservative level allows for the greater protection of everyone—adults, children, and even unborn babies. In six random samples, Vital Choice sockeye salmon, for example, tested at .02 ppm for mercury and no detect for PCBs (detection threshold .02 ppm). To learn more, visit About Seafood at www.vitalchoice.com.

A Word About Antibiotics

According to the Union of Concerned Scientists (www.ucsusa.org), more than 68 percent of all seafood consumed in the United States is imported, and most of it is industrially produced. Many of these commodities are farm-raised and often involve little oversight regarding antibiotic drug use. While the U.S. government has standards that should ban imports with high levels of antibiotics in seafood, there is essentially no enforcement. Farmed salmon have more antibiotics administered by weight than any other form of livestock.

Here is additional information from the U.S. government on the mercury issue:

United States Department of Health and Human Services and the Environmental Protection Agency

What You Need to Know About Mercury in Fish and Shellfish
2004 EPA and FDA

Advice for:

Women who might become pregnant

Women who are pregnant

Nursing mothers

Young children

Fish and shellfish are an important part of a healthy diet. Fish and shellfish contain high-quality protein and other essential nutrients, are low in saturated fat, and contain omega-3 fatty acids. A well-balanced diet that includes a variety of fish and shellfish can contribute to heart health and children's proper growth and development. So, women and young children in particular should include fish or shellfish in their diets due to the many nutritional benefits.

However, nearly all fish and shellfish contain traces of mercury. For most people, the risk from mercury by eating fish and shellfish is not a health concern. Yet, some fish and shellfish contain higher levels of mercury that may harm an unborn baby or young child's developing nervous system. The risks from mercury in fish and shellfish depend on the amount of fish and shellfish eaten and the levels of mercury in the fish and shellfish. Therefore, the Food and Drug Administration (FDA) and the Environmental Protection Agency (EPA) are advising women who may become pregnant, pregnant women, nursing mothers, and young children to avoid some types of fish and eat fish and shellfish that are lower in mercury.

By following these three recommendations for selecting and eating fish or shellfish, women and young children will receive the benefits of eating fish and shellfish and be confident that they have reduced their exposure to the harmful effects of mercury.

1. Do not eat shark, swordfish, king mackerel, or tilefish because they contain high levels of mercury.

2. Eat up to 12 ounces (two average meals) a week of a variety of fish and shellfish that are lower in mercury. Five of the most commonly eaten fish that are low in mercury are shrimp, canned light tuna, **salmon,** pollock, and catfish.

   ◆ Another commonly eaten fish, albacore ("white") tuna has more mercury than canned light tuna. So, when choosing your two meals of fish and shellfish, you may eat up to 6 ounces (one average meal) of albacore tuna per week.

3. Check local advisories about the safety of fish caught by family and friends in your local lakes, rivers, and coastal areas. If no advice is available, eat up to 6 ounces (one average meal) per week of fish you catch from local waters, but don't consume any other fish during that week.

Follow these same recommendations when feeding fish and shellfish to your young child, but serve smaller portions.

Frequently Asked Questions About Mercury in Fish and Shellfish

1. "What is mercury and methyl mercury?"

   Mercury occurs naturally in the environment and can also be released into the air through industrial pollution. Mercury falls from the air and can accumulate in streams and oceans and is turned into methyl mercury in the water. It is this type of mercury that can be harmful to your unborn baby and young child. Fish absorb the methyl mercury as they feed in these waters and so it builds up in them. It builds up more in some types of fish and shellfish than others, depending on what the fish eat, which is why the levels vary.

2. "I'm a woman who could have children but I'm not pregnant, so why should I be concerned about methyl mercury?"

   If you regularly eat types of fish that are high in methyl mercury, it can accumulate in your bloodstream over time. Methyl mercury is removed from the body naturally, but it may take more than a year for the levels to drop significantly. Thus, it may be present in a woman even before she becomes pregnant. This is the reason why women who are trying to become pregnant should also avoid eating certain types of fish.

3. "Is there methyl mercury in all fish and shellfish?"

   Nearly all fish and shellfish contain traces of methyl mercury. However, larger fish that have lived longer have the highest levels of methyl mercury because they've had more time to accumulate it. These large fish (swordfish, shark, king mackerel, and tilefish) pose the greatest risk. Other types of fish and shellfish may be eaten in the amounts recommended by FDA and EPA.

4. "I don't see the fish I eat in the advisory. What should I do?"

   If you want more information about the levels in the various types of fish you eat, see the FDA food safety website at www.cfsan.fda.gov/~frf/sea-mehg.html or the EPA website at www.epa.gov/ost/fish.

5. "What about fish sticks and fast-food sandwiches?"

   Fish sticks and fast-food sandwiches are commonly made from fish that are low in mercury.

6. "The advice about canned tuna is in the advisory, but what's the advice about tuna steaks?"

Because tuna steak generally contains higher levels of mercury than canned light tuna, when choosing your two meals of fish and shellfish, you may eat up to 6 ounces (one average meal) of tuna steak per week.

7. "Where do I get information about the safety of fish caught recreationally by family or friends?"

Before you go fishing, check your Fishing Regulations Booklet for information about recreationally caught fish. You can also contact your local health department for information about local advisories. You need to check local advisories because some kinds of fish and shellfish caught in your local waters may have higher or much lower than average levels of mercury. This depends on the levels of mercury in the water in which the fish are caught. Those fish with much lower levels may be eaten more frequently and in larger amounts.

For further information about the risks of mercury in fish and shellfish call the U.S. Food and Drug Administration's food information line toll-free at 888-SAFEFOOD or visit the FDA's Food Safety website at www.cfsan.fda.gov/seafood1.html.

For further information about the safety of locally caught fish and shellfish, visit the Environmental Protection Agency's Fish Advisory website at www.epa.gov/ost/fish or contact your state or local health department. A list of state or local health department contacts is available at www.epa.gov/ost/fish. Click on Federal, State, and Tribal Contacts. For information on the EPA's actions to control mercury, visit the EPA's mercury website at www.epa.gov/mercury. This document is available at www.cfsan.fda.gov/~dms/admehg3.html.

As you can see from the comprehensive documentations, wild salmon is a safe, healthy food choice. For more information log on to www.cfsan.fda.gov/seafood1.html or www.vitalchoice.com.

Average Mercury Levels in Common Seafood

Courtesy of www.vitalchoice.com

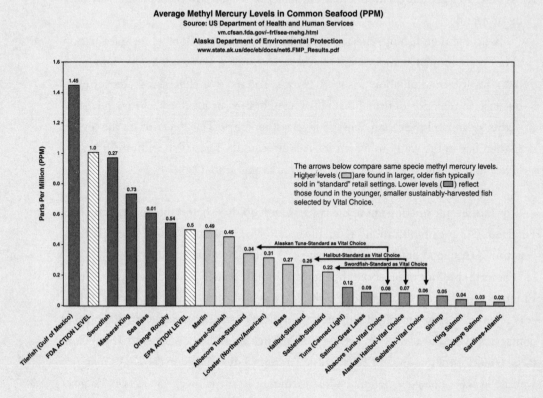

Average Methyl Mercury Levels in Common Seafood (PPM)
Source: US Department of Health and Human Services
vm.cfsan.fda.gov/~frf/sea-mehg.html
Alaska Department of Environmental Protection
www.state.ak.us/dec/eb/docs/net6.FMP_Results.pdf

The arrows below compare same specie methyl mercury levels. Higher levels (□)are found in larger, older fish typically sold in "standard" retail settings. Lower levels (■) reflect those found in the younger, smaller sustainably-harvested fish selected by Vital Choice.

Resource Guide

Cosmeceutical Skin Care

Antioxidant, anti-inflammatory topical products–formulated by Dr. Perricone to help maintain firmness and tone even during weight loss–are available at:

- N.V. Perricone, M.D., Ltd., at 888-823-7837 or www.nvperriconemd.com
- N.V. Perricone, M.D., Ltd., Flagship Store at 791 Madison Avenue (corner of 67th Street), New York, NY
- Nordstrom
- Sephora
- Saks Fifth Avenue
- Neiman Marcus
- Henri Bendel
- Clyde's on Madison (926 Madison Avenue at 74th Street, New York, NY)
- Bloomingdale's
- Belk's
- Parisian

NUTRITIONAL SUPPLEMENTS

Polysaccharide Peptide Food™

This anti-inflammatory, antiaging beverage mix and food topping is custom manufactured to Dr. Perricone's specifications.

- N.V. Perricone, M.D., Ltd., at 888-823-7837 or www.nvperriconemd.com
- N.V. Perricone, M.D., Ltd., Flagship Store at 791 Madison Avenue (at 67th Street), New York, NY
- All retail partners listed above

Weight Management Supplements

Weight Management Program™ supplements formulated by Dr. Perricone are available at:

- N.V. Perricone, M.D., Ltd., at 888-823-7837 or www.nvperriconemd.com
- N.V. Perricone M.D. Ltd., Flagship Store at 791 Madison Avenue (at 67th Street), New York, NY
- All retail partners listed on page 233

Antiaging, Anti-inflammatory Supplements

Skin and Total Body Nutritional Supplements™ formulated by Dr. Perricone are available at:

- N.V. Perricone, M.D., Ltd., at 888-823-7837 or www.nvperriconemd.com
- N.V. Perricone M.D. Ltd., Flagship Store at 791 Madison Avenue (at 67th Street), New York, NY
- All retail partners listed on page 233
- Optimum Health International (Stephen Sinatra, M.D.) at 800-228-1507 or www.opthealth.com
- Life Extension Foundation at 800-544-4440 or www.lef.org

Astaxanthin (Highly Potent Antioxidant Found in Salmon and Marine Zooplankton)

- N.V. Perricone, M.D., Ltd., at 888-823-7837 or www.nvperriconemd.com
- All retail partners listed on page 233

Omega-3 Fish Oil

- N.V. Perricone, M.D., Ltd., at 888-823-7837 or www.nvperriconemd.com
- N.V. Perricone M.D. Ltd., Flagship Store at 79 Madison Avenue (at 67th Street) New York, NY
- Vital Choice Seafood at 800-608-4825 or www.vitalchoice.com
- All retail partners listed on page 233
- Optimum Health International, at 800-228-1507 or www.opthealth.com

Maitake D-Fraction and SX-Fraction Extract

◆ N.V. Perricone, M.D., Ltd., at 888-823-7837 or www.nvperriconemd.com
◆ Maitake Products, Inc., at 800-747-7418 or www.maitake.com

Maitake Magic (Freedom Press), Harry Preuss, M.D., www.amazon.com

Anti-inflammatory Herbal Supplements

New Chapter, Inc. markets potent anti-inflammatory herbal extracts. The company employs CO_2, water, and alcohol extraction to yield an unusually broad spectrum of active constituents from ginger, turmeric, rosemary, and other anti-inflammatory herbs. www.new-chapter.com or 800-543-7279.

DR. PERRICONE'S SUPERFOODS

Wild Alaskan Salmon and Seafood; Wild Organic Berries

Vital Choice Seafood offers wild-harvested fresh-frozen fish (salmon, sablefish, sardines, tuna, and halibut) and fresh-frozen organic blueberries, raspberries, and strawberries. Their fish are flash-frozen on the boats and packed in dry ice for delivery via FedEx or UPS. Compared with farmed salmon, wild Alaskan salmon offers greater purity and a healthier fatty-acid profile (less saturated fat; higher ratio of omega-3 fatty-acids to omega-6 fatty acids). www.vitalchoice.com or 800-608-4825.

Açaí (Amazonian Fruit High in Antioxidants)

Açaí fruit has more antioxidants than wild blueberries, pomegranates, or red wine; it also contains essential omega-3s (healthy fats), amino acids, calcium, and fiber. Sambazon brand açaí concentrate, smoothies, and supplements can be ordered from www.sambazon.com and are sold nationwide at Whole Foods Market and Wild Oats stores. A portion of all profits from product sales are reinvested into environmental and social programs within the Amazon to promote biodiversity and reduce poverty.

Avocados

The California Avocado Board offers recipes and health information at www.avocado.org and www.spectrumorganics.com.

Beans and Lentils (Organic and Heirloom)

◆ Bob's Red Mill sells direct at www.bobsredmill.com or 800-349-2173.

◆ Diamond Organics, Inc., sells direct at www.diamondorganics.com or 888-674-2642.

◆ Westbrae Natural sells through retailers. For locations, go to www.westbrae.com/products/index.html or call 800-434-4246.

Chili Peppers

◆ Diamond Organics, Inc. at www.diamondorganics.com or call 888-674-2642.

Cinnamon Extract

◆ New Chapter, Inc. makes Cinnamonforce, a high-potency CO_2 extract of the two species of cinnamon. Go to www.new-chapter.com/product/supercritical.lasso or www.new-chapter.com/buy/index.html (retail outlets) or call 800-543-7279.

◆ Natrol offers a standard cinnamon extract at www.natrol.com or 800-262-8765.

Grain-Free Crackers

◆ Foods Alive Organic Golden Flax Crackers at www.foodsalive.com

Flaxseed

◆ Bob's Red Mill at www.bobsredmill.com

Grains (Full Selection, Including Whole Organic Buckwheat and Oats)

◆ Bob's Red Mill at www.bobsredmill.com

Grass-Fed and Organic Meats

◆ Eatwild.com is an information clearinghouse for consumers seeking grass-fed and organic beef, lamb, goat, bison, poultry, and dairy products. The site's principal researcher and writer is Jo Robinson, the *New York Times* bestselling author of *Pasture Perfect* and *The Omega Diet* (written with renowned fatty-acid researcher Dr. Artemis Simopoulos). www.eatwild.com.

Kefir and Yogurt

◆ Helios Nutrition is a small organic dairy in Sauk Centre, Minnesota, that makes several flavors of organic kefir with added FOS (prebiotic polysaccharide). Locate retail outlets at 888-3-HELIOS or www.heliosnutrition.com/html/where_to_buy.html.

◆ Lifeway Foods of Morton Grove, Illinois, makes kefir and related products with national distribution. www.lifeway.net/

◆ Stonyfield Farm Yogurt (natural and organic varieties) is available at many food markets. See the store locator at www.stonyfield.com/StoreLocator/.

◆ Horizon Organic yogurt is available at many food markets. See the store locator at www.horizonorganic.com/findingproducts/index.html.

Luo Han Kao (Uniquely High in Antioxidants)

◆ Longjiang River Health Products, LLC, One Bridge Street, Irvington-On-Hudson, NY 10533. info@longjiangriver.com or 888-916-1688.

Pomegranate Juice and Concentrate (Extremely High in Antioxidants)

◆ POM Wonderful at 310-966-5800 or www.pomwonderful.com
◆ Also available at supermarkets and natural food stores

Organic Extra Virgin Olive Oil

◆ N.V. Perricone, M.D., Ltd., Flagship Store at 791 Madison Avenue (corner of 67th Street), New York, NY.

◆ Soler Romero Organic Extra Virgin Olive Oil (superior quality and flavor) www.odysseyfoods.com or 360-825-2814

◆ International Olive Oil Council at www.internationaloliveoil.org/

◆ California Olive Growers at www.oliveoilsource.com/oliveoildr.htm

Retail Outlets (Natural and Organic Foods)

◆ Diamond Organics, Inc. is a direct-to-consumer Internet retailer of certified-organic fruits, vegetables, nuts, grains, beans, spices, and more. www.diamondorganics.com or 1-888-674-2642.

◆ Whole Foods Market (www.wholefoods.com) and Wild Oats (www.wildoats.com). These are the two largest natural foods supermarket chains in the United States. Both sell every kind of fresh food (e.g., fish, meat, poultry, fruits, vegetables, eggs, cheese, kefir, yogurt), frozen food, and grocery item (bulk grains, nuts, seeds, beans, cereals, canned goods, sauces, condiments) you would find in a regular supermarket, but without synthetic additives or sweeteners. Their selections include many certified organic foods, as well as natural health- and body-care items (supplements, kefir, yogurt, etc.). Log on to their website to find a store near you.

Sprouts: Information and Supplies

◆ The International Sprout Growers Association (ISGA) is the professional association of sprout growers and companies that supply products and services to the sprout industry. Visit their website for outstanding information, recipes, and health notes (www.isga-sprouts.org).

◆ "Sproutman" Steve Meyerowitz is one of the world's leading proponents of do-it-yourself sprouting. 413-528-5200, www.sproutman.com, or P.O. Box 1100, Great Barrington, MA 01230.

Tea

◆ The Yau Hing Company offers high-quality teas (green, white, and black) with high antioxidant (polyphenol) content, at 415-395-0868 or www.YHTEAS.com.

Pure Water

◆ From the Fiji Islands, this natural artesian water is filtered for centuries through volcanic geology. Available nationwide and at www.fijiwater.com.

◆ Poland Spring Natural Spring Water is a pure and natural spring water from Maine available nationwide or at www.polandspring.com.

EXERCISE

Outstanding information on the benefits and types of exercise, including drawings:

◆ President's Council on Physical Fitness (PCPFS), www.fitness.gov

◆ The National Institute of Aging, www.niapublications.org

NUTRITION AND HEALTH INFORMATION

Cancer-preventing Foods

◆ The American Institute for Cancer Research. www.aicr.org

Life Extension Foundation

◆ Current scientific news and information on food and nutritional supplements, including the latest on the weight-loss benefits of sesame seed. An outstanding website! www.lef.org.

Fats of Life and PUFA Newsletter

◆ An excellent website and e-mail newsletter concerning essential fatty acids. www.fatsoflife.com

Food and Nutrition Information Center (USDA)

◆ www.nal.usda.gov/fnic/

Outstanding Health and Nutrition Information

◆ WholeHealthMD.com is American WholeHealth Networks' award-winning Complementary and Alternative Medicine (CAM) education website. www.wholehealthmd.com.

Glycemic Index (University of Sydney)

◆ General information on the glycemic index, and a searchable foods database. www.glycemicindex.com.

The European Food Information Council

◆ EUFIC, is a nonprofit organization that provides science-based information on food and food-related topics to the media, health and nutrition professionals, educators, and opinion leaders. www.eufic.org.

Mercola.com

◆ Information from Joseph Mercola, M.D., concerning conventional and alternative medicine, and the health implications of various foods and supplements (vitamins, minerals, fatty acids, nutraceuticals, phytoceuticals). www.mercola.com.

National Institutes of Health (NIH)

◆ Links to all NIH centers at www.nih.gov/icd/

Nutrition Source at Harvard School of Public Health

◆ www.hsph.harvard.edu/nutritionsource/index.html

Seafood Safety

◆ Environmental Working Group at www.ewg.org/issues/mercury/20050314/index.php (Mercury issues) and www.ewg.org/reports/farmedPCBs/part2.php (farmed salmon issues)

◆ Oceans Alive at www.oceansalive.org/eat.cfm?subnav=healthalerts

◆ U.S Food and Drug Administration Center for Food Safety at www.cfsan.fda.gov/~frf/sea-mehg.html

◆ U.S. Environmental Protection Agency (EPA) at www.epa.gov/ost/fish.and www.epa.gov/mercury

◆ Vital Choice Seafood at www.vitalchoice.com/purity.cfm and www.vitalchoice.com/newsletter_index2.cfm

Soy Foods

◆ Indiana Soybean Development Council (Stevens & Associates) at www.soyfoods.com

◆ Weston A. Price Foundation soy critiques at www.westonaprice.org/soy/index.html and www.westonaprice.org/mythstruths/mtsoy.html

Sweeteners (Noncaloric, Nonglycemic)

◆ www.holisticmed.com/sweet/

◆ Stevia at www.stevia.net

◆ ZSweet natural sugar substitute at www.zsweet.com

◆ Luo Han Kao at www.longjiangriver.com

World's Healthiest Foods (George Mateljan Foundation)

◆ Detailed information on healthful whole foods (e.g., fruits, vegetables, nuts, seeds, beans, grains, herbs, spices), including many recipes. www.whfoods.com.

Wheat and Gluten Allergies

◆ www.celiac.com

RECIPES

◆ For flavorful, healthful recipes, as featured in *The Perricone Weight-Loss Diet*, we recommend *Stop the Clock! Cooking* by Cheryl Forberg, R.D. www.amazon.com

References

CHAPTER 1: GETTING STARTED

- Brown CD, Higgins M, Donato KA, Rohde RC, Garrison R, Obarzanek E, Ernst ND, Horan M. Body mass index and prevalence of hypertension and dyslipidemia. Obesity Res. 2000;8(9):605–619.
- Calle EE, Rodriguez C, Walker-Thurmond K, Thun MJ. Overweight, obesity, and mortality from cancer in a prospectively studied cohort of U.S. adults. N Engl J Med. 2003;348(17):1625–1638.
- Clinical Guidelines on the Identification, Evaluation, and Treatment of Overweight and Obesity in Adults–The Evidence Report. National Institutes of Health. Obesity Res. 1998;6 (suppl)2:51S-209S.
- Flegal KM, Carroll MD, Kuczmarski RJ, Johnson CL. Overweight and obesity in the United States: Prevalence and trends, 1960–1994. Int J Obesity. 1998;22:39–47.
- Flegal KM, Carroll MD, Ogden CL, Johnson CL. Prevalence and trends in obesity among US adults, 1999–2000. JAMA. 2002;288:1723–1727.
- Fontaine KR, Redden DT, Wang C, Westfall AO, Allison DB. Years of life lost due to obesity. JAMA. 2003;289(2):187–93.
- International Obesity TaskForce. Obesity in Europe–3 International Obesity TaskForce March 2005. Accessed online June 20, 2005 at www.iotf.org/media/europrev.htm
- Kuczmarski RJ, Flegal KM. Criteria for definition of overweight in transition: Background and recommendations for the United States. Am J Clin Nutr. 2000;72:1074–1081.
- Kuczmarski RJ, Ogden CL, Guo SS, et al. 2000 CDC growth charts for the United States: Methods and development. National Center for Health Statistics. Vital Health Statistics 11(246). 2002.

- Mokdad AH, Bowman BA, Ford ES, Vinicor F, Marks JS, Koplan JP. The continuing epidemics of obesity and diabetes in the United States. JAMA. 2001;286(10):1195–1200.

- Mokdad AH, Ford ES, Bowman BA, Dietz WH, Vinicor F, Bales VS, Marks JS. Prevalence of obesity, diabetes, and obesity-related health risk factors, 2001. JAMA. 2003;289(1):76–79.

- Ogden CL, Flegal KM, Carroll MD, Johnson CL. Prevalence and trends in overweight among US children and adolescents, 1999–2000. JAMA. 2002;288:1728–1732.

- Pastor PN, Makuc DM, Reuben C, Xia H. Chartbook on Trends in the Health of Americans. Health, United States, 2002. Hyattsville, MD: National Center for Health Statistics, 2002.

- U.S. Department of Health and Human Services. The Surgeon General's Call to Action to Prevent and Decrease Overweight and Obesity. Washington D.C., 2001.

- Weight-control Information Network. Statistics Related to Overweight and Obesity. Accessed online June 20, 2005 at win.niddk.nih.gov/statistics/

CHAPTER 2: THE INFLAMMATION–AGING–DISEASE–OBESITY CONNECTION AND CHAPTER 3: BREAKING THE INFLAMMATION–FAT CONNECTION

- Adler V, Yin Z, Tew KD, Ronai Z. Role of redox potential and reactive oxygen species in stress signaling. Oncogene. 1999 Nov 1;18(45):6104–11. Review.

- Allen RG, Tresini M. Oxidative stress and gene regulation. Free Radic Biol Med. 2000 Feb 1;28(3):463–99. Review.

- Bailey AJ. Molecular mechanisms of aging in connective tissues. Mech Aging Dev. 2001 May 31;122(7):735–55. Review.

- Bastard JP, Vidal H, Jardel C, Bruckert E, Robin D, Vallier P, Blondy P, Turpin G, Forest C, Hainque B. Subcutaneous adipose tissue expression of plasminogen activator inhibitor-1 gene during very low calorie diet in obese subjects. Int J Obes Relat Metab Disord. 2000 Jan;24(1):70–4.

- Black PH, Garbutt LD. Stress, inflammation and cardiovascular disease. J Psychosom Res. 2002 Jan;52(1):1–23.

- Brod SA. Unregulated inflammation shortens human functional longevity. Inflamm Res. 2000 Nov;49(11):561–70. Review.

- Bruunsgaard H, Pedersen M, Pedersen BK. Aging and proinflammatory cytokines. Curr Opin Hematol. 2001 May;8(3):131–6. Review.

- Cai D, Yuan M, Frantz DF, Melendez PA, Hansen L, Lee J, Shoelson SE. Local and systemic insulin resistance resulting from hepatic activation of IKK-beta and NF-kappaB. Nat Med. 2005 Feb;11(2):183–90. Epub 2005 Jan 30.

- Camhi SL, Lee P, Choi AM. The oxidative stress response. New Horiz. 1995 May;3(2):170–82. Review.

- Cefalu WT, Bell-Farrow AD, Wang ZQ, Sonntag WE, Fu MX, Baynes JW, Thorpe SR. Caloric restriction decreases age-dependent accumulation of the glycoxidation products, N epsilon-(carboxymethyl)lysine and pentosidine, in rat skin collagen. J Gerontol A Biol Sci Med Sci. 1995 Nov;50(6):B337–41.

- Christman JW, Blackwell TS, Juurlink BH. Redox regulation of nuclear factor kappa B: therapeutic potential for attenuating inflammatory responses. Brain Pathol. 2000 Jan;10(1):153–62. Review.

- Clement K, Viguerie N, Poitou C, Carette C, Pelloux V, Curat CA, Sicard A, Rome S, Benis A, Zucker JD, Vidal H, Laville M, Barsh GS, Basdevant A, Stich V, Cancello R, Langin D. Weight loss regulates inflammation-related genes in white adipose tissue of obese subjects. FASEB J. 2004 Nov;18(14):1657–69.

- Du Y, Chen X, Wei X, Bales KR, Berg DT, Paul SM, Farlow MR, Maloney B, Ge YW, Lahiri DK. NF-kappaB mediates amyloid beta peptide-stimulated activity of the human apolipoprotein E gene promoter in human astroglial cells. Brain Res Mol Brain Res. 2005 May 20;136(1–2):177–88.

- Engeli S, Feldpausch M, Gorzelniak K, Hartwig F, Heintze U, Janke J, Mohlig M, Pfeiffer AF, Luft FC, Sharma AM. Association between adiponectin and mediators of inflammation in obese women. Diabetes. 2003 Apr;52(4):942–7.

- Finkel T. Redox-dependent signal transduction. FEBS Lett. 2000 Jun 30;476(1–2):52–4. Review.

- Franceschi C, Bonafe M, Valensin S, Olivieri F, De Luca M, Ottaviani E, De Benedictis G. Inflamm-aging. An evolutionary perspective on immunosenescence. Ann N Y Acad Sci 2000 Jun;908:244–54.

- Franceschi C, et al. Neuroinflammation and the genetics of Alzheimer's disease: the search for a pro-inflammatory phenotype. Aging (Milano). 2001 Jun;13(3):163–70. Review.

- Franceschi C, et al. The network and the remodeling theories of aging: historical background and new perspectives. Exp Gerontol. 2000 Sep;35(6–7):879–96. Review.

- Fu MX, et al. Glycation, glycoxidation, and cross-linking of collagen by glucose. Kinetics, mechanisms, and inhibition of late stages of the Maillard reaction. Diabetes. 1994 May;43(5):676–83.

- Gamaley IA, Klyubin IV. Roles of reactive oxygen species: signaling and regulation of cellular functions. Int Rev Cytol. 1999;188:203–55. Review.

- Garaulet M, Viguerie N, Porubsky S, Klimcakova E, Clement K, Langin D, Stich V. Adiponectin gene expression and plasma values in obese women during very-low-calorie diet. Relationship with cardiovascular risk factors and insulin resistance. J Clin Endocrinol Metab. 2004 Feb;89(2):756–60.

- Ghanim H, Aljada A, Hofmeyer D, Syed T, Mohanty P, Dandona P. Circulating mononuclear cells in the obese are in a proinflammatory state. Circulation. 2004 Sep 21;110(12):1564–71. Epub 2004 Sep 13.

- Gius D, Botero A, Shah S, Curry HA. Intracellular oxidation/reduction status in the regulation of transcription factors NF-kappaB and AP-1. Toxicol Lett. 1999 Jun 1;106(2–3):93–106. Review.

- Hirose N, et al. [Suggestions from a centenarian study–aging and inflammation] Nippon Ronen Igakkai Zasshi. 2001 Mar;38(2):121–4. Review. Japanese.

- Esposito K, Marfella R, Ciotola M, Di Palo C, Giugliano F, Giugliano G, D'Armiento M, D'Andrea F, Giugliano D. Effect of a Mediterranean-style diet on endothelial dysfunction and markers of vascular inflammation in the metabolic syndrome: a randomized trial. JAMA. 2004;292:1440–1446.

- Lavrovsky Y, Chatterjee B, Clark RA, Roy AK. Role of redox-regulated transcription factors in inflammation, aging and age-related diseases. Exp Gerontol. 2000 Aug;35(5):521–32. Review.

- Lehrke M, Reilly MP, Millington SC, Iqbal N, Rader DJ, Lazar MA. An inflammatory cascade leading to hyperresistinemia in humans. PLoS Med. 2004 Nov;1(2):e45. Epub 2004 Nov 30.

- Lin Y, Rajala MW, Berger JP, Moller DE, Barzilai N, Scherer PE. Hyperglycemia-induced production of acute phase reactants in adipose tissue. J Biol Chem. 2001 Nov 9;276(45):42077–83.

- Maher P, Schubert D. Signaling by reactive oxygen species in the nervous system. Cell Mol Life Sci. 2000 Aug;57(8–9):1287–305. Review.
- Norlin S, Ahlgren U, Edlund H. Nuclear factor-[kappa]B activity in [beta]-cells is required for glucose-stimulated insulin secretion. Diabetes. 2005 Jan;54(1):125–32.
- Nose K. Role of reactive oxygen species in the regulation of physiological functions. Biol Pharm Bull. 2000 Aug;23(8):897–903. Review.
- Ozcan U, Cao Q, Yilmaz E, Lee AH, Iwakoshi NN, Ozdelen E, Tuncman G, Gorgun C, Glimcher LH, Hotamisligil GS. Endoplasmic reticulum stress links obesity, insulin action, and type 2 diabetes. Science. 2004 Oct 15;306(5695):457–61.
- Pedersen SB, Borglum JD, Kristensen K, Norrelund H, Otto J, Jorgensen L, Richelsen B. Regulation of uncoupling protein (UCP) 2 and 3 in adipose and muscle tissue by fasting and growth hormone treatment in obese humans. Int J Obes Relat Metab Disord. 2000 Aug;24(8):968–75.
- Redonnet A, Bonilla S, Noel-Suberville C, Pallet V, Dabadie H, Gin H, Higueret P. Relationship between peroxisome proliferator-activated receptor gamma and retinoic acid receptor alpha gene expression in obese human adipose tissue. Int J Obes Relat Metab Disord. 2002 Jul;26(7):920–7.
- Ribot J, Rantala M, Kesaniemi YA, Palou A, Savolainen MJ. Weight loss reduces expression of SREBP1c/ADD1 and PPARgamma2 in adipose tissue of obese women. Pflugers Arch. 2001 Jan;441(4):498–505.
- Roy AK. Transcription factors and aging. Mol Med. 1997 Aug;3(8):496–504. Review.
- Sen CK, Packer L. Antioxidant and redox regulation of gene transcription. FASEB J. 1996 May;10(7):709–20. Review.
- Sharma AM. Regulation of 11beta-HSD genes in human adipose tissue: influence of central obesity and weight loss. Obes Res. 2004 Jan;12(1):9–17.
- Shi C, Zhao X, Wang X, Andersson R. Role of nuclear factor-kappaB, reactive oxygen species and cellular signaling in the early phase of acute pancreatitis. Scand J Gastroenterol. 2005 Jan;40(1):103–8.
- Shoelson SE, Lee J, Yuan M. Inflammation and the IKK beta/I kappa B/NF-kappa B axis in obesity- and diet-induced insulin resistance. Int J Obes Relat Metab Disord. 2003 Dec;27 Suppl 3:S49–52. Review.
- Slater AF, Nobel CS, Orrenius S. The role of intracellular oxidants in apoptosis. Biochim Biophys Acta. 1995 May 24;1271(1):59–62. Review.

- Spiteller G. Peroxidation of linoleic acid and its relation to aging and age dependent diseases. Mech Aging Dev. 2001 May 31;122(7):617–57. Review.

- Thannickal VJ, Fanburg BL. Reactive oxygen species in cell signaling. Am J Physiol Lung Cell Mol Physiol. 2000 Dec;279(6):L1005–28. Review.

- Vidal-Puig AJ, Considine RV, Jimenez-Linan M, Werman A, Pories WJ, Caro JF, Flier JS. Peroxisome proliferator-activated receptor gene expression in human tissues. Effects of obesity, weight loss, and regulation by insulin and glucocorticoids. J Clin Invest. 1997 May 15;99(10):2416–22.

- Wilhelm J. Metabolic aspects of membrane lipid peroxidation. Acta Univ Carol Med Monogr. 1990;137:1–53. Review.

- Yim MB, Yim HS, Lee C, Kang SO, Chock PB. Protein glycation: creation of catalytic sites for free radical generation. Ann N Y Acad Sci. 2001 Apr;928:48–53.

- Zs-Nagy I, Cutler RG, Semsei I. Dysdifferentiation hypothesis of aging and cancer: a comparison with the membrane hypothesis of aging. Ann N Y Acad Sci. 1988;521:215–25. Review.

- Zs-Nagy I, Semsei I. Centrophenoxine increases the rates of total and mRNA synthesis in the brain cortex of old rats: an explanation of its action in terms of the membrane hypothesis of aging. Exp Gerontol. 1984;19(3):171–8.

- Zs-Nagy I. The membrane hypothesis of aging: its relevance to recent progress in genetic research. J Mol Med. 1997 Oct;75(10):703–14. Review.

- Zs-Nagy I. The role of membrane structure and function in cellular aging: a review. Mech Aging Dev. 1979 Feb;9(3–4):237–46. Review.

CHAPTER 4: THE OMEGA-3 WEIGHT LOSS-MIRACLE

- Barak Y, Liao D, He W, et al. Effects of peroxisome proliferator-activated receptor [delta] on placentation, adiposity and colorectal cancer. Proc Nat Acad Sci USA. 2002;99:303–308.

- Browning LM. N-3 polyunsaturated fatty acids, inflammation and obesity-related disease. Proc Nutr Soc. 2003 May;62(2):447–53. Review.

- Chen H, Charlat O, Tartaglia LA, et al. Evidence that the diabetes gene encodes the leptin receptor: identification of a mutation in the leptin receptor gene in db/db mice. Cell. 1996;84:491–495.

- Clarke SD. Polyunsaturated fatty acid regulation of gene transcription: a mechanism to improve energy balance and insulin resistance. Br J Nutr. 2000 Mar;83 Suppl 1:S59–66. Review.

♦ Clarke SD. Polyunsaturated fatty acid regulation of gene transcription: a mechanism to improve energy balance and insulin resistance. Br J Nutr. 2000 Mar;83 Suppl 1:S59–66. Review.

♦ Clarke SD, Thuillier P, Baillie RA, Sha X. Peroxisome proliferator-activated receptors: a family of lipid-activated transcription factors. Am J Clin Nutr. 1999 Oct;70(4):566–71. Review. Biochimie 1998;79:95–99.

♦ Delarue J, LeFoll C, Corporeau C, Lucas D. N-3 long chain polyunsaturated fatty acids: a nutritional tool to prevent insulin resistance associated to type 2 diabetes and obesity? Reprod Nutr Dev. 2004 May-Jun;44(3):289–99. Review. "n-3 LC-PUFA stimulate fatty acid oxidation in the liver (via the activation of peroxisome proliferator activated receptor alpha (PPAR-alpha)."

♦ Delarue J, LeFoll C, Corporeau C, Lucas D. N-3 long chain polyunsaturated fatty acids: a nutritional tool to prevent insulin resistance associated to type 2 diabetes and obesity? Reprod Nutr Dev. 2004 May-Jun;44(3):289–99. Review.

♦ Duplus E, Glorian M, Forest C. Fatty acid regulation of gene transcription. J Biol Chem. 2000 Oct 6;275(40):30749–52. Review.

♦ Field FJ, Born E, Murthy S, Mathur SN. Polyunsaturated fatty acids decrease the expression of sterol regulatory element-binding protein-1 in CaCo-2 cells: effect on fatty acid synthesis and triacylglycerol transport. Biochem J. 2002 Dec; 15(368)(Pt 3):855–64.

♦ Forman BM, Chen J, Evans RM. Hypolipidemic drugs, polyunsaturated fatty acids and eicosanoids are ligands for peroxisome proliferator-activated receptors a and [delta]. Proc Nat Acad Sci USA. 1997;94:4312–4317.

♦ Garvey WT. The role of uncoupling protein 3 in human physiology. J Clin Invest. 2003 Feb;111(4):438–41.

♦ Jump DB, Clarke SD. Regulation of gene expression by dietary fat. Annu Rev Nutr. 1999;19:63–90. Review.

♦ Kuriki K, Nagaya T, Tokudome Y, Imaeda N, Fujiwara N, Sato J, Goto C, Ikeda M, Maki S, Tajima K, Tokudome S. Plasma concentrations of (n-3) highly unsaturated fatty acids are good biomarkers of relative dietary fatty acid intakes: a cross-sectional study. J Nutr. 2003 Nov;133(11):3643–50.

♦ Lee C-H, Olson P, Evans RM. Minireview: lipid metabolism, metabolic diseases, and peroxisome proliferator-activated receptors. Endocrinology. 2003; 144:2201–2207.

◆ Li H, Ruan XZ, Powis SH, Fernando R, Mon WY, Wheeler DC, Moorhead JF, Varghese Z. EPA and DHA reduce LPS-induced inflammation responses in HK-2 cells: evidence for a PPAR-gamma-dependent mechanism. Kidney Int. 2005 Mar;67(3):867–74. "Our data demonstrate that both EPA and DHA down-regulate LPS-induced activation of NF-kappaB via a PPAR-gamma-dependent pathway in HK-2 cells. These results suggest that PPAR-gamma activation by EPA and DHA may be one of the underlying mechanisms for the beneficial effects of fish oil."

◆ Lovejoy JC. The influence of dietary fat on insulin resistance. Curr Diab Rep. 2002 Oct;2(5):435–40. Review.

◆ Manco M, Calvani M, Mingrone G. Effects of dietary fatty acids on insulin sensitivity and secretion. Diabetes Obes Metab. 2004 Nov;6(6):402–13. Review.

◆ Massiera F, Saint-Marc P, Seydoux J, Murata T, Kobayashi T, Narumiya S, Guesnet P, Amri EZ, Negrel R, Ailhaud G. Arachidonic acid and prostacyclin signaling promote adipose tissue development: a human health concern? J Lipid Res. 2003 Feb;44(2):271–9. Epub 2002 Nov 04.

◆ Mori TA, Bao DQ, Burke V, Puddey IB, Watts GF, Beilin LJ. Dietary fish as a major component of a weight-loss diet: effect on serum lipids, glucose, and insulin metabolism in overweight hypertensive subjects. Am J Clin Nutr. 1999 Nov;70(5):817–25.

◆ Mori TA, Burke V, Puddey IB, Shaw JE, Beilin LJ. Effect of fish diets and weight loss on serum leptin concentration in overweight, treated-hypertensive subjects. J Hypertens. 2004 Oct;22(10):1983–90.

◆ Mishra A, Chaudhary A, Sethi S. Oxidized omega-3 fatty acids inhibit NF-kappaB activation via a PPARalpha-dependent pathway. Arterioscler Thromb Vasc Biol. 2004 Sep;24(9):1621–7. Epub 2004 Jul 1.

◆ Oliver WR Jr, Shenk JL, Snaith MR, et al. A selective peroxisome proliferator-activated receptor delta agonist promotes reverse cholesterol transport. Proc Nat Acad Sci USA. 2001;98:5306–5311.

◆ Oudart H, Groscolas R, Calgari C, Nibbelink M, Leray C, Le Maho Y, Malan A. Brown fat thermogenesis in rats fed high-fat diets enriched with n-3 polyunsaturated fatty acids. Int J Obes Relat Metab Disord. 1997 Nov;21(11):955–62.

◆ Pischon T, Hankinson SE, Hotamisligil GS, Rifai N, Willett WC, Rimm EB. Habitual dietary intake of n-3 and n-6 fatty acids in relation to inflammatory markers among US men and women. Circulation. 2003 Jul 15;108(2):155–60. Epub 2003 Jun 23.

◆ Power GW, Newsholme EA. Dietary fatty acids influence the activity and metabolic control of mitochondrial carnitine palmitoyltransferase I in rat heart and skeletal muscle. J Nutr. 1997 Nov;127(11):2142–50.

◆ Rivellese AA, Lilli S. Quality of dietary fatty acids, insulin sensitivity and type 2 diabetes. Biomed Pharmacother. 2003 Mar;57(2):84–7. Review.

◆ Sessler AM, Ntambi JM. Polyunsaturated fatty acid regulation of gene expression. J Nutr. 1998 Jun;128(6):923–6. Review.

◆ Simopoulos AP. Omega-3 fatty acids in inflammation and autoimmune diseases. J Am Coll Nutr. 2002 Dec;21(6):495–505.

◆ Sulzle A, Hirche F, Eder K. Thermally oxidized dietary fat upregulates the expression of target genes of PPAR alpha in rat liver. J Nutr. 2004 Jun;134(6):1375–83.

◆ Ukropec J, Reseland JE, Gasperikova D, Demcakova E, Madsen L, Berge RK, Rustan AC, Klimes I, Drevon CA, Sebokova E. The hypotriglyceridemic effect of dietary n-3 FA is associated with increased beta-oxidation and reduced leptin expression. Lipids. 2003 Oct;38(10):1023–9.

◆ Vessby B, Unsitupa M, Hermansen K, Riccardi G, Rivellese AA, Tapsell LC, Nalsen C, Berglund L, Louheranta A, Rasmussen BM, Calvert GD, Maffetone A, Pedersen E, Gustafsson IB, Storlien LH; KANWU Study. Substituting dietary saturated for monounsaturated fat impairs insulin sensitivity in healthy men and women: The KANWU Study. Diabetologia. 2001 Mar;44(3):312–9.

◆ Wang Y-X, Lee C-H, Tiep S, et al. Peroxisome-proliferator [delta] activates fat metabolism to prevent obesity. Cell. 2003;113:159–170.

◆ Wang YX, Lee CH, Tiep S, Yu RT, Ham J, Kang H, Evans RM. Peroxisome-proliferator-activated receptor delta activates fat metabolism to prevent obesity. Cell. 2003 Apr 18;113(2):159–70. "Our findings suggest that PPARdelta serves as a widespread regulator of fat burning and identify PPARdelta as a potential target in the treatment of obesity and its associated disorders."

◆ Wolf, G. The Function of the Nuclear Receptor Peroxisome Proliferator-activated Receptor Delta in Energy Homeostasis. Nutrition Reviews, Nov 2003.

- Yamauchi T, Waki H, Kamon J, Murakami K, Motojima K, Komeda K, Miki H, Kubota N, Terauchi Y, Tsuchida A, Tsuboyama-Kasaoka N, Yamauchi N, Ide T, Hori W, Kato S, Fukayama M, Akanuma Y, Ezaki O, Itai A, Nagai R, Kimura S, Tobe K, Kagechika H, Shudo K, Kadowaki T. Inhibition of RXR and PPARgamma ameliorates diet-induced obesity and type 2 diabetes. J Clin Invest. 2001 Oct;108(7):1001–13. "Our data suggested that appropriate functional antagonism of PPARgamma/RXR may be a logical approach to protection against obesity and related diseases such as type 2 diabetes."

- Zhao Y, Joshi-Barve S, Barve S, Chen LH. Eicosapentaenoic acid prevents LPS-induced TNF-alpha expression by preventing NF-kappaB activation. J Am Coll Nutr. 2004 Feb;23(1):71–8. "CONCLUSIONS: The results suggest that suppression of the TNF-alpha expression by EPA is partly attributed to its inhibitory effect on NF-kappaB activation. EPA appears to prevent NF-kappaB activation by preventing the phosphorylation of IkappaB-alpha."

CHAPTER 5: STEP ONE: THE TOP 10 FOOD GROUPS FOR PERMANENT WEIGHT LOSS

#1: Rich Fish

- Browning LM. N-3 polyunsaturated fatty acids, inflammation and obesity-related disease. Proc Nutr Soc. 2003 May;62(2):447–53. Review.

- Clarke SD, Thuillier P, Baillie RA, Sha X. Peroxisome proliferator-activated receptors: a family of lipid-activated transcription factors. Am J Clin Nutr. 1999 Oct;70(4):566–71. Review. Biochimie 1998;79:95–99

- Clarke SD. Polyunsaturated fatty acid regulation of gene transcription: a mechanism to improve energy balance and insulin resistance. Br J Nutr. 2000 Mar;83 Suppl 1:S59–66. Review.

- Clarke SD. Polyunsaturated fatty acid regulation of gene transcription: a mechanism to improve energy balance and insulin resistance. Br J Nutr. 2000 Mar;83 Suppl 1:S59–66. Review.

- Delarue J, LeFoll C, Corporeau C, Lucas D. N-3 long chain polyunsaturated fatty acids: a nutritional tool to prevent insulin resistance associated to type 2 diabetes and obesity? Reprod Nutr Dev. 2004 May-Jun;44(3):289–99. Review.

♦ Duplus E, Glorian M, Forest C. Fatty acid regulation of gene transcription. J Biol Chem. 2000 Oct 6;275(40):30749–52. Review.

♦ Field FJ, Born E, Murthy S, Mathur SN. Polyunsaturated fatty acids decrease the expression of sterol regulatory element-binding protein-1 in CaCo-2 cells: effect on fatty acid synthesis and triacylglycerol transport. Biochem J. 2002 Dec 15; 368(Pt 3):855–64.

♦ Garvey WT. The role of uncoupling protein 3 in human physiology. J Clin Invest. 2003 Feb;111(4):438–41.

♦ Jump DB, Clarke SD. Regulation of gene expression by dietary fat. Annu Rev Nutr. 1999;19:63–90. Review.

♦ Kuriki K, Nagaya T, Tokudome Y, Imaeda N, Fujiwara N, Sato J, Goto C, Ikeda M, Maki S, Tajima K, Tokudome S. Plasma concentrations of (n-3) highly unsaturated fatty acids are good biomarkers of relative dietary fatty acid intakes: a cross-sectional study. J Nutr. 2003 Nov;133(11):3643–50.

♦ Li H, Ruan XZ, Powis SH, Fernando R, Mon WY, Wheeler DC, Moorhead JF, Varghese Z. EPA and DHA reduce LPS-induced inflammation responses in HK-2 cells: evidence for a PPAR-gamma-dependent mechanism. Kidney Int. 2005 Mar;67(3):867–74.

♦ Lovejoy JC. The influence of dietary fat on insulin resistance. Curr Diab Rep. 2002 Oct;2(5):435–40. Review.

♦ Manco M, Calvani M, Mingrone G. Effects of dietary fatty acids on insulin sensitivity and secretion. Diabetes Obes Metab. 2004 Nov;6(6):402–13. Review.

♦ Massiera F, Saint-Marc P, Seydoux J, Murata T, Kobayashi T, Narumiya S, Guesnet P, Amri EZ, Negrel R, Ailhaud G. Arachidonic acid and prostacyclin signaling promote adipose tissue development: a human health concern? J Lipid Res. 2003 Feb;44(2):271–9. Epub 2002 Nov 04.

♦ Mishra A, Chaudhary A, Sethi S. Oxidized omega-3 fatty acids inhibit NF-kappaB activation via a PPARalpha-dependent pathway. Arterioscler Thromb Vasc Biol. 2004 Sep;24(9):1621–7. Epub 2004 Jul 1.

♦ Mori TA, Bao DQ, Burke V, Puddey IB, Watts GF, Beilin LJ. Dietary fish as a major component of a weight-loss diet: effect on serum lipids, glucose, and insulin metabolism in overweight hypertensive subjects. Am J Clin Nutr. 1999 Nov;70(5):817–25.

◆ Mori TA, Burke V, Puddey IB, Shaw JE, Beilin LJ. Effect of fish diets and weight loss on serum leptin concentration in overweight, treated-hypertensive subjects. J Hypertens. 2004 Oct;22(10):1983–90.

◆ Oudart H, Groscolas R, Calgari C, Nibbelink M, Leray C, Le Maho Y, Malan A. Brown fat thermogenesis in rats fed high-fat diets enriched with n-3 polyunsaturated fatty acids. Int J Obes Relat Metab Disord. 1997 Nov;21(11):955–62.

◆ Pischon T, Hankinson SE, Hotamisligil GS, Rifai N, Willett WC, Rimm EB. Habitual dietary intake of n-3 and n-6 fatty acids in relation to inflammatory markers among US men and women. Circulation. 2003 Jul 15;108(2):155–60. Epub 2003 Jun 23.

◆ Power GW, Newsholme EA. Dietary fatty acids influence the activity and metabolic control of mitochondrial carnitine palmitoyltransferase I in rat heart and skeletal muscle. J Nutr. 1997 Nov;127(11):2142–50.

◆ Rivellese AA, Lilli S. Quality of dietary fatty acids, insulin sensitivity and type 2 diabetes. Biomed Pharmacother. 2003 Mar;57(2):84–7. Review.

◆ Sessler AM, Ntambi JM. Polyunsaturated fatty acid regulation of gene expression. J Nutr. 1998 Jun;128(6):923–6. Review.

◆ Simopoulos AP.Omega-3 fatty acids in inflammation and autoimmune diseases. J Am Coll Nutr. 2002 Dec;21(6):495–505.

◆ Sulzle A, Hirche F, Eder K. Thermally oxidized dietary fat upregulates the expression of target genes of PPAR alpha in rat liver. J Nutr. 2004 Jun;134(6):1375–83.

◆ Ukropec J, Reseland JE, Gasperikova D, Demcakova E, Madsen L, Berge RK, Rustan AC, Klimes I, Drevon CA, Sebokova E. The hypotriglyceridemic effect of dietary n-3 FA is associated with increased beta-oxidation and reduced leptin expression. Lipids. 2003 Oct;38(10):1023–9.

◆ Vessby B, Unsitupa M, Hermansen K, Riccardi G, Rivellese AA, Tapsell LC, Nalsen C, Berglund L, Louheranta A, Rasmussen BM, Calvert GD, Maffetone A, Pedersen E, Gustafsson IB, Storlien LH; KANWU Study. Substituting dietary saturated for monounsaturated fat impairs insulin sensitivity in healthy men and women: The KANWU Study. Diabetologia. 2001 Mar;44(3):312–9.

◆ Zhao Y, Joshi-Barve S, Barve S, Chen LH. Eicosapentaenoic acid prevents LPS-induced TNF-alpha expression by preventing NF-kappaB activation. J Am Coll Nutr. 2004 Feb;23(1):71–8.

#2: Fruits

◆ Crespy, V et al. Bioavailability of phloretin and phloridzin in rats. Nutri. 2001:131:3227–3230.

◆ Ding M, Lu Y, Bowman L, Huang C, Leonard S, Wang L, Vallyathan V, Castranova V, Shi X. Inhibition of AP-1 and neoplastic transformation by fresh apple peel extract. J Biol Chem. 2004 Mar 12;279(11):10670–6. Epub 2003 Dec 9.

◆ Feng R, Bowman LL, Lu Y, Leonard SS, Shi X, Jiang BH, Castranova V, Vallyathan V, Ding M. Blackberry extracts inhibit activating protein 1 activation and cell transformation by perturbing the mitogenic signaling pathway. Nutr Cancer. 2004;50(1):80–9.

◆ Fujioka K, Greenway F, Sheard J. Effects of grapefruit and grapefruit products on weight and metabolic syndrome. Oral Presentation, American Chemical Society 228th National Meeting, Philadelphia, August 24–25, 2004.

◆ Hongu, M et al. Na(+)-glucose cotransporter inhibitors as antidiabetic agents. II. Synthesis and structure-activity relationships of 4'-dehydroxyphlorizin derivatives. Chem Pharm Bull (Tokyo). 1998;46:22–33.

◆ Knekt, P et al. Flavonoid intake and risk of chronic diseases. Am J Clin Nutr. 2002;76:560–568.

◆ Rolls B, Barnett RA. The Volumetrics Weight-Control Plan, New York: Harper Torch, 2003.

◆ Tiwary, CM, Ward, JA, Jackson, BA. J Am Coll Nutr. 1997;16(5)423–428.

◆ Wang SY, Feng R, Bowman L, Penhallegon R, Ding M, Lu Y. Antioxidant activity in lingonberries (Vaccinium vitis-idaea L.) and its inhibitory effect on activator protein-1, nuclear factor-kappaB, and mitogen-activated protein kinases activation. J Agric Food Chem. 2005 Apr 20;53(8):3156–66.

◆ Wang SY, Feng R, Lu Y, Bowman L, Ding M. Inhibitory effect on activator protein-1, nuclear factor-kappaB, and cell transformation by extracts of strawberries (Fragaria x ananassa Duch.). J Agric Food Chem. 2005 May 18;53(10):4187–4193.

#3: Fats from Fruits

◆ Bell EA, Rolls BJ. Energy density of foods affects energy intake across multiple levels of fat content in lean and obese women. Am J Clin Nutr 2001;73(6):1010–1018.

◆ Crozier G, Bois-Joyeux B, Chanex M, et al. Overfeeding with medium-chain triglycerides in the rat. Metabolism 1987;36:807–814.

◆ Endres J, Barter S, Theodora P, Welch P., Soy-enhanced lunch acceptance by preschoolers. J Am Diet Assoc. 2003 Mar;103(3):346–51.

◆ Franz MJ, et al. Evidence-Based Nutrition Principles and Recommendations for the Treatment and Prevention of Diabetes and Related Complications (Technical Review). Diabetes Care 2002;25:148–198.

◆ Griswold KE, Apgar GA, et al. Effectiveness of short-term feeding strategies for altering conjugated linoleic acid content of beef. J Animal Sci, 2003 Jul;81(7):1862–71.

◆ Hill JO, Peters JC, Yang D, Sharp T, Kaler M, Abumrad NN, Greene HL. Thermogenesis in humans during overfeeding with medium-chain triglycerides. Metabolism. July.1989;38(7):641–8.

◆ Kabara JJ. Health oils from the tree of life (nutritional and health aspects of coconut oil.) Indian Coconut Journal. 2000;31(8):2–8.

◆ Mayer B, Kalus U, Grigorov A, Pindur G, Jung F, Radtke H, Bachmann K, Mrowietz C, Koscielny J, Wenzel E, Kiesewetter H. Effects of an onion-olive oil maceration product containing essential ingredients of the Mediterranean diet on blood pressure and blood fluidity. Arzneimittelforschung. 2001 Feb;51(2):104–11.

◆ Madigan C, Ryan M, Owens D, Collins P, Tomkin GH. Dietary unsaturated fatty acids in type 2 diabetes: higher levels of postprandial lipoprotein on a linoleic acid-rich sunflower oil diet compared with an oleic acid-rich olive oil diet. Diabetes Care. 2000 Oct;23(10):1472–7.

◆ Rocca AS, LaGreca J, Kalitsky J, Brubaker PL. Monounsaturated fatty acid diets improve glycemic tolerance through increased secretion of glucagon-like peptide-1. Endocrinology. 2001 Mar;142(3):1148–55.

◆ Rodriguez-Villar C, Manzanares JM, Casals E, Perez-Heras A, Zambon D, Gomis R, Ros E. High-monounsaturated fat, olive oil-rich diet has effects similar to a high-carbohydrate diet on fasting and postprandial state and metabolic profiles of patients with type 2 diabetes. Metabolism. 2000 Dec;49(12):1511–7.

◆ Rolls B, Barnett RA. The Volumetrics Weight-Control Plan. New York: Harper Torch, 2003.

◆ Rolls BJ. Presentation, 2004 Annual Scientific Meeting of the North American Association for the Study of Obesity.

◆ Russell R. What the Bible Says About Healthy Living. Ventura, CA: Regal Books 1996, 125.

◆ Scollan ND, Enser M, et al. Effects of including a ruminally protected lipid supplement in the diet on the fatty acid composition of beef muscle. Br J Nutr. 2003 Sep;90(3):709–16.

◆ Seaton TB, Welles SL, Warenko MK, et al. Thermic effects of medium-chain and long-chain triglycerides in man. Am J Clin Nutr. 1986;44:630–634.

◆ See, MT, Odle, J. Effect of dietary fat source, level, and feeding interval on pork fatty acid composition. 1998–2000 Departmental Report, Department of Animal Science, ANS Report No. 248–North Carolina State University.

◆ St-Onge MP, Ross R, Parsons WD, Jones PJ. Medium-chain triglycerides increase energy expenditure and decrease adiposity in overweight men. Obes Res. 2003 Mar;11(3):395–402.

◆ Taubes G. What If It Were All a Big Fat Lie! New York Times, 7 July 2002.

◆ Trinidad TP, Valdez DH, Loyola AS, Mallillin AC, Askali FC, Castillo JC, Masa DB. Glycaemic index of different coconut (Cocos nucifera)-flour products in normal and diabetic subjects. Br J Nutr. 2003 Sep;90(3):551–6.

◆ U.S. Department of Health and Human Services. Centers for Disease Control. Obesity Still on the Rise, New Data Show. Accessed online October 8, 2002 at www.cdc.gov/nchs/releases/02news/obesityonrise.htm

◆ Votruba SB, Atkinson RL, Schoeller DA. Prior exercise increases dietary oleate, but not palmitate oxidation. Obesity Research 2003;11(12):1509–1518.

#4: Spice Things Up

◆ Anderson RA, Broadhurst CL, Polansky MM, Schmidt WF, Khan A, Flanagan VP, Schoene NW, Graves DJ. Isolation and characterization of polyphenol type-A polymers from cinnamon with insulin-like biological activity. J Agric Food Chem. 2004 Jan 14;52(1):65–70.

◆ Arun N, Nalini N. Efficacy of turmeric on blood sugar and polyol pathway in diabetic albino rats. Plant Foods Hum Nutr. 2002 Winter;57(1):41–52.

◆ Bahijri SM, Mufti AM. Beneficial effects of chromium in people with type 2 diabetes, and urinary chromium response to glucose load as a possible indicator of status. Biol Trace Elem Res. 2002 Feb;85(2):97–109.

◆ Broadhurst CL, Polansky MM, Anderson RA. Insulin-like biological activity of culinary and medicinal plant aqueous extracts in vitro. J Agric Food Chem. 2000 Mar;48(3):849–52.

◆ Broca C, Breil V, Cruciani-Guglielmacci C, Manteghetti M, Rouault C, Derouet M, Rizkalla S, Pau B, Petit P, Ribes G, Ktorza A, Gross R, Reach G, Taouis M. Insulinotropic agent ID-1101 (4-hydroxyisoleucine) activates insulin signaling in rat. Am J Physiol Endocrinol Metab. 2004 Sep;287(3):E463–71. Epub 2004 Apr 13.

◆ Devi BA, Kamalakkannan N, Prince PS. Supplementation of fenugreek leaves to diabetic rats. Effect on carbohydrate metabolic enzymes in diabetic liver and kidney. Phytother Res. 2003 Dec;17(10):1231–3.

◆ Guan X, Matte JJ, Ku PK, Snow JL, Burton JL, Trottier NL. High chromium yeast supplementation improves glucose tolerance in pigs by decreasing hepatic extraction of insulin. J Nutr. 2000 May;130(5):1274–9.

◆ Gupta A, Gupta R, Lal B. Effect of Trigonella foenum-graecum (fenugreek) seeds on glycaemic control and insulin resistance in type 2 diabetes mellitus: a double blind placebo controlled study. J Assoc Physicians India. 2001 Nov;49:1057–61.

◆ Imparl-Radosevich J, Deas S, Polansky MM, Baedke DA, Ingebritsen TS, Anderson RA, Graves DJ. Regulation of PTP-1 and insulin receptor kinase by fractions from cinnamon: implications for cinnamon regulation of insulin signaling. Horm Res. 1998 Sep;50(3):177–82.

◆ Jarvill-Taylor KJ, Anderson RA, Graves DJ. A hydroxychalcone derived from cinnamon functions as a mimetic for insulin in 3T3-L1 adipocytes. J Am Coll Nutr. 2001 Aug;20(4):327–36.

◆ Khan A, Safdar M, Ali Khan MM, Khattak KN, Anderson RA. Cinnamon improves glucose and lipids of people with type 2 diabetes. Diabetes Care. 2003 Dec;26(12):3215–8.

◆ Kubo K, Aoki H, Nanba H. Anti-diabetic activity present in the fruit body of Grifola frondosa (Maitake). I. Biol Pharm Bull. 1994 Aug;17(8):1106–10.

◆ Manohar V, Talpur NA, Echard BW, Lieberman S, Preuss HG. Effects of a water-soluble extract of maitake mushroom on circulating glucose/insulin concentrations in KK mice. Diabetes Obes Metab. 2002 Jan;4(1):43–8.

♦ Nishiyama T, Mae T, Kishida H, Tsukagawa M, Mimaki Y, Kuroda M, Sashida Y, Takahashi K, Kawada T, Nakagawa K, Kitahara M. Curcuminoids and sesquiterpenoids in turmeric (Curcuma longa L.) suppress an increase in blood glucose level in type 2 diabetic KK-Ay mice. J Agric Food Chem. 2005 Feb 23;53(4):959–63.

♦ Qin B, Nagasaki M, Ren M, Bajotto G, Oshida Y, Sato Y. Cinnamon extract prevents the insulin resistance induced by a high-fructose diet. Horm Metab Res. 2004 Feb;36(2):119–25.

♦ Qin B, Nagasaki M, Ren M, Bajotto G, Oshida Y, Sato Y. Cinnamon extract (traditional herb) potentiates in vivo insulin-regulated glucose utilization via enhancing insulin signaling in rats. Diabetes Res Clin Pract. 2003 Dec;62(3):139–48.

♦ Ruby BC, Gaskill SE, Slivka D, Harger SG. The addition of fenugreek extract (Trigonella foenum-graecum) to glucose feeding increases muscle glycogen resynthesis after exercise. Amino Acids. 2005 Feb;28(1):71–6. Epub 2004 Dec 2.

♦ Sridhar SB, Sheetal UD, Pai MR, Shastri MS. Preclinical evaluation of the antidiabetic effect of Eugenia jambolana seed powder in streptozotocin-diabetic rats. Braz J Med Biol Res. 2005 Mar;38(3):463–8. Epub 2005 Mar 8.

♦ Thakran S, Siddiqui MR, Baquer NZ. Trigonella foenum graecum seed powder protects against histopathological abnormalities in tissues of diabetic rats. Mol Cell Biochem. 2004 Nov;266(1–2):151–9.

#5: Heat Things Up

♦ Buiatti E, Palli D, Decarli A, et al. A case-control study of gastric cancer and diet in Italy. Int J Cancer. 1989;44:611–6.

♦ Chaiyata P, Puttadechakum S, Komindr S. Effect of chili pepper (Capsicum frutescens) ingestion on plasma glucose response and metabolic rate in Thai women. J Med Assoc Thai. 2003 Sep;86(9):854–60.

♦ Dickerson C. Neuropeptide regulation of proinflammatory cytokine responses. J Leukoc Biol 1998 May;63(5):602–5.

♦ Edwards SJ, et al. Spicy meal disturbs sleep: an effect of thermoregulation? Int J Psychophysiol. 1992 Sep;13(2):97–100.

- Kobayashi A. Capsaicin activates heat loss and heat production simultaneously and independently in rats. Am J Physiol. 1998 Jul;275(1 Pt 2):R92–8.

- Kwak JY. A capsaicin-receptor antagonist, capsazepine, reduces inflammation-induced hyperalgesic responses in the rat: evidence for an endogenous capsaicin-like substance. Neuroscience. 1998 Sep;86(2):619–26.

- Lim K, Yoshioka M, Kikuzato S, Kiyonaga A, Tanaka H, Shindo M, Suzuki M. Dietary red pepper ingestion increases carbohydrate oxidation at rest and during exercise in runners. Med Sci Sports Exerc. 1997 Mar;29(3):355–61.

- Lopez-Carrillo L, Avila M, Dubrow R. Chili pepper consumption and gastric cancer in Mexico: A case-control study. Amer J Epidem. 1994;139:263–71.

- Matsumoto T, Miyawaki C, Ue H, Yuasa T, Miyatsuji A, Moritani T. Effects of capsaicin-containing yellow curry sauce on sympathetic nervous system activity and diet-induced thermogenesis in lean and obese young women. J Nutr Sci Vitaminol (Tokyo). 2000 Dec;46(6):309–15.

- Mitchell JA. Role of nitric oxide in the dilator actions of capsaicin-sensitive nerves in the rabbit coronary circulation. Neuropeptides. 1997 Aug;31(4):333–8.

- Nelson AG. The effect of capsaicin on the thermal and metabolic responses of men exposed to 38 degrees C for 120 minutes. Wilderness Environ Med. 2000 Fall;11(3):152–6.

- Ohnuki K, Niwa S, Maeda S, Inoue N, Yazawa S, Fushiki T. CH-19 sweet, a non-pungent cultivar of red pepper, increased body temperature and oxygen consumption in humans. Biosci Biotechnol Biochem. 2001 Sep;65(9):2033–6.

- Pacach AS. The effect of capsaicin on orally-measured body temperature. Accessed online May 15, 2005 at www.usc.edu/CSSF/History/2004/Projects/J1421.pdf

- Siften DW (ed). Physicians' Desk Reference for Nonprescription Drugs. Montvale, NJ: Medical Economics, 1998, 790–1.

- Surh YJ, Lee SS. Capsaicin in hot chili pepper: Carcinogen, co-carcinogen or anticarcinogen? Food Chem Toxic. 1996;34:313–6.

- Yoshioka M, Doucet E, Drapeau V, Dionne I, Tremblay A. Combined effects of red pepper and caffeine consumption on 24 h energy balance in subjects given free access to foods. Br J Nutr. 2001 Feb;85(2):203–11.

- Yoshioka M, Imanaga M, Ueyama H, Yamane M, Kubo Y, Boivin A, St-Amand J, Tanaka H, Kiyonaga A. Maximum tolerable dose of red pepper decreases fat intake independently of spicy sensation in the mouth. Br J Nutr. 2004 Jun;91(6):991–5.

- Yoshioka M, Lim K, Kikuzato S, Kiyonaga A, Tanaka H, Shindo M, Suzuki M. Effects of red-pepper diet on the energy metabolism in men. J Nutr Sci Vitaminol (Tokyo). 1995 Dec;41(6):647–56.

- Yoshioka M, St-Pierre S, Drapeau V, Dionne I, Doucet E, Suzuki M, Tremblay A. Effects of red pepper on appetite and energy intake. Br J Nutr. 1999 Aug;82(2):115–23.

- Yoshioka M, St-Pierre S, Suzuki M, Tremblay A. Effects of red pepper added to high-fat and high-carbohydrate meals on energy metabolism and substrate utilization in Japanese women. Br J Nutr. 1998 Dec;80(6):503–10.

#6 Seeds and Nuts

- Edwards JU. Flaxseed: Agriculture to Health, FN-596, October 2003. Accessed online June 20, 2005 at www.ext.nodak.edu/extpubs/yf/foods/fn596.htm

- Garcia-Lorda P, Megias Rangil I, Salas-Salvado J. Nut consumption, body weight and insulin resistance. Eur J Clin Nutr. 2003 Sep;57 Suppl 1:S8–11. Review.

- Kontush A, Spranger T, Reich A, Baum K, Beisiegel U. Lipophilic antioxidants in blood plasma as markers of atherosclerosis: the role of alpha-carotene and gamma-tocopherol. Atherosclerosis. 1999 Jun;144(1):117–22.

- Megias-Rangil I, Garcia-Lorda P, Torres-Moreno M, Bullo M, Salas-Salvado J. [Nutrient content and health effects of nuts.] Arch Latinoam Nutr. 2004 Jun;54(2 Suppl 1):83–6. Spanish.

- Minamiyama Y, Takemura S, Yoshikawa T, Okada S. Fermented grain products, production, properties and benefits to health. Pathophysiology. 2003 Oct;9(4):221–7.

- Prasad K. Hypocholesterolemic and antiatherosclerotic effect of flax lignan complex isolated from flaxseed. Atherosclerosis. 2005 Apr;179(2):269–75. Epub 2005 Jan 26.

- Qidwai W, Alim SR, Dhanani RH, et al. Use of folk remedies among patients in Karachi Pakistan. J Ayub Med Coll Abbottabad. 2003 Apr;15(2):31–3.

- Sabate J. Nut consumption and body weight. Am J Clin Nutr. 2003 Sep;78(3 Suppl):647S-650S. Review.

- Takeuchi H, Mooi LY, Inagaki Y, He P. Hypoglycemic effect of a hot-water extract from defatted sesame (Sesamum indicum L.) seed on the blood glucose level in genetically diabetic KK-Ay mice. Biosci Biotechnol Biochem. 2001 Oct;65(10):2318–21.
- Yamashita K, Nohara Y, Katayama K, Nami ki M. Sesame seed lignans and gamma-tocopherol act synergistically to produce vitamin E activity in rats. J Nutr. 1992;122(12):2440–6.

#7: Beans and Lentils

- Boivin M, Flourie B, Rizza RA, et al. Gastrointestinal and metabolic effects of amylase inhibition in diabetics. Gastroenterology. 1988;94:387–94.
- Boivin M, Zinsmeister AR, Go VL, DiMagno EP. Effect of a purified amylase inhibitor on carbohydrate metabolism after a mixed meal in healthy humans. Mayo Clin Proc. 1987;62:249–55.
- Bo-Linn GW, Santa Ana CA, Morawski SG, Fordtran JS. Starch blockers– their effect on calorie absorption from a high-starch meal. N Engl J Med. 1982;307:1413–6.
- Brugge WR, Rosenfeld MS. Impairment of starch absorption by a potent amylase inhibitor. Am J Gastroenterol. 1987;82:718–22.
- Carlson GL, Li BU, Bass P, Olsen WA. A bean alpha-amylase inhibitor formulation (starch blocker) is ineffective in man. Science. 1983;219:393–5.
- Englyst HN, Veenstra J, Hudson GJ. Measurement of rapidly available glucose (RAG) in plant foods: a potential in vitro predictor of the glycaemic response. Br J Nutr. 1996 Mar;75(3):327–37.
- Garrow JS, Scott PF, Heels S, et al. A study of "starch blockers" in man using 13C-enriched starch as a tracer. Hum Nutr Clin Nutr. 1983;37:301–5.
- Granfeldt Y, Drews A, Bjorck I. Arepas made from high amylose corn flour produce favorably low glucose and insulin responses in healthy humans. J Nutr. 1995 Mar;125(3):459–65.
- Higgins JA, Higbee DR, Donahoo WT, Brown IL, Bell ML, Bessesen DH. Resistant starch consumption promotes lipid oxidation. Nutr Metab (Lond). 2004 Oct 6;1(1):8.

- Higgins JA. Resistant STARch: metabolic effects and potential health benefits. J AOAC Int. 2004 May-Jun;87(3):761–8. Review.

- Hollenbeck CB, Coulston AM, Quan R, et al. Effects of a commercial starch blocker preparation on carbohydrate digestion and absorption: in vivo and in vitro studies. Am J Clin Nutr. 1983;38:498–503.

- Holt PR, Thea D, Yang MY, Kotler DP. Intestinal and metabolic responses to an alpha-glucosidase inhibitor in normal volunteers. Metabolism. 1988;37:1163–70.

- Kendall CW, Emam A, Augustin LS, Jenkins DJ. Resistant STARches and health. J AOAC Int. 2004 May-Jun;87(3):769–74. Review.

- Lankisch M, Layer P, Rizza RA, DiMagno EP. Acute postprandial gastrointestinal and metabolic effects of wheat amylase inhibitor (WAI) in normal, obese, and diabetic humans. Pancreas. 1998 Aug;17(2):176–81.

- Robertson MD, Currie JM, Morgan LM, Jewell DP, Frayn KN. Prior short-term consumption of resistant STARch enhances postprandial insulin sensitivity in healthy subjects. Diabetologia. 2003 May;46(5):659–65. Epub 2003 Apr 24.

- Udani J, Hardy M, Madsen DC. Blocking carbohydrate absorption and weight loss: a clinical trial using phase 2 brand proprietary fractionated white bean extract. Altern Med Rev. 2004 Mar;9(1):63–9.

#8: Low-fat Dairy

- Barba G, Troiano E, Russo P, Venezia A, Siani A. Inverse association between body mass and frequency of milk consumption in children. J Nutr. 2005 Jan;93(1):15–9.

- Barr SI. Increased dairy product or calcium intake: is body weight or composition affected in humans? J Nutr. 2003 Jan;133(1):245S-248S. Review.

- Bianchi G, Marzocchi R, Agostini F, Marchesini G. Update on nutritional supplementation with branched-chain amino acids. Curr Opin Clin Nutr Metab Care. 2005 Jan;8(1):83–7. Review.

- Bowen J, Noakes M, Clifton PM. Effect of calcium and dairy foods in high protein, energy-restricted diets on weight loss and metabolic parameters in overweight adults. Int J Obes Relat Metab Disord. 2005 Feb 15; [Epub ahead of print].

- Carruth BR, Skinner JD. The role of dietary calcium and other nutrients in modeCW rating body fat in preschool children. Int J Obes Relat Metab Disord. 2001 Apr;25(4):559–66.

- Chan GM, Hoffman K, McMurry M. Effects of dairy products on bone and body composition in pubertal girls. J Pediatr. 1995 Apr;126(4):551–6.

- Cheirsilp B, Shimizu H, Shioya S. Enhanced kefiran production by mixed culture of Lactobacillus kefiranofaciens and Saccharomyces cerevisiae. J Biotechnol. 2003 Jan 9;100(1):43–53.

- Davies KM, Heaney RP, Recker RR, Lappe JM, Barger-Lux MJ, Rafferty K, Hinders S. Calcium intake and body weight. J Clin Endocrinol Metab. 2000 Dec;85(12):4635–8.

- Davies KM, Heaney RP, Recker RR, et al. Calcium intake and body weight J Clin Endocrinol Metab. 2000; 85:4635–4638.

- Elmer GW, Surawicz CM, McFarland LV. Biotherapeutic agents. JAMA. 1996;275:870–6.

- Frengova GI, Simova ED, Beshkova DM, Simov ZI. Exopolysaccharides produced by lactic acid bacteria of kefir grains. Z Naturforsch [C]. 2002 Sep-Oct;57(9–10):805–10.

- Gluck U, Gebbers JO. Ingested probiotics reduce nasal colonization with pathogenic bacteria (Staphylococcus aureus, Streptococcus pneumoniae, and beta-hemolytic streptococci). Am J Clin Nutr. 2003 Feb;77(2):517–20.

- Gunther CW, Legowski PA, Lyle RM, McCabe GP, Eagan MS, Peacock M, Teegarden D. Dairy products do not lead to alterations in body weight or fat mass in young women in a 1-y intervention. Am J Clin Nutr. 2005 Apr;81(4):751–6.

- Heaney RP, Davies KM, Barger-Lux MJ. Calcium and weight: clinical studies. J Am Coll Nutr. 2002 Apr;21(2):152S-155S. Review.

- Heaney RP. Normalizing calcium intake: projected population effects for body weight. J Nutr. 2003; 133:268S-270S.

- Hilton E, Isenberg HD, Alperstein P, et al. Ingestion of yogurt containing Lactobacillus acidophilus as prophylaxis for candidal vaginitis. Ann Intern Med. 1992;116:353–7.

- Kailasapathy K, Chin J. Survival and therapeutic potential of probiotic organisms with reference to Lactobacillus acidophilus and Bifidobacterium spp. Immunol Cell Biol. 2000 Feb;78(1):80–8. Review.

- Lin YC, Lyle RM, McCabe LD, McCabe GP, Weaver CM, Teegarden D. Dairy calcium is related to changes in body composition during a two-year exercise intervention in young women. J Am Coll Nutr. 2000 Nov-Dec;19(6):754–60.

- Mack DR, Lebel S. Role of probiotics in the modulation of intestinal infections and inflammation. Curr Opin Gastroenterol. 2004 Jan;20(1):22–6.

- Marteau P, Seksik P, Lepage P, Dore J. Cellular and physiological effects of probiotics and prebiotics. Mini Rev Med Chem. 2004 Oct;4(8):889–96. Review.

- Morris K, Wang Y, Kim SY, Moustaid-Moussa N. Dietary and hormonal regulation of the mammalian fatty acid synthase gene. In: Moustaid-Moussa N, Berdanier CD, (eds). Nutrient-Gene Interactions in Health and Disease. Boca Raton, FL: CRC Press, 2001.

- Mullally MM, Meisel H, FitzGerald RJ. Identification of a novel angiotensin-l-converting enzyme inhibitory peptide corresponding to a tryptic fragment of bovine beta-lactoglobulin. FEBS Lett. 1997;402:99–101.

- Nikolaeva TN, Zorina VV, Bondarenko VM. [Immunostimulating and anti-carcinogenic activity of the normal intestinal lactoflora.] Eksp Klin Gastroenterol. 2004;(4):39–43, 109. Review. Russian.

- Nikolaeva TN, Zorina VV, Bondarenko VM. [The role of cytokines in the immunoreactivity modulation with bacteria of the Lactobacillus genus.] Zh Mikrobiol Epidemiol Immunobiol. 2004 Nov-Dec;(6):101–6. Review. Russian.

- Noverr MC, Huffnagle GB. Does the microbiota regulate immune responses outside the gut? Trends Microbiol. 2004 Dec;12(12):562–8. Review.

- Papakonstantinou E, Flatt WP, Huth PJ, Harris RB. High dietary calcium reduces body fat content, digestibility of fat, and serum vitamin D in rats. Obes Res. 2003 Mar;11(3):387–94.

- Perdigon G, Alvarez S, Rachid M, Aguero G, Gobbato N. Immune system stimulation by probiotics. J Dairy Sci. 1995 Jul;78(7):1597–606. Review.

- Perdigon G, Maldonado Galdeano C, Valdez JC, Medici M. Interaction of lactic acid bacteria with the gut immune system. Eur J Clin Nutr. 2002 Dec;56 Suppl 4:S21–6.

- Perdigon G, Vintini E, Alvarez S, Medina M, Medici M. Study of the possible mechanisms involved in the mucosal immune system activation by lactic acid bacteria. J Dairy Sci. 1999 Jun;82(6):1108–14.

- Pihlanto-Leppala A, Koskinen P, Piilola K, Tupasela T, Korhonen H. Angiotensin I-converting enzyme inhibitory properties of whey protein digests: concentration and characterization of active peptides. J Dairy Res. 2000;67:53–64.

- Reid G, Millsap K, Bruce AW. Implantation of Lactobacillus casei var rhamnosus into vagina. Lancet. 1994;344:1229.

- Shah NP. Effects of milk-derived bioactives: an overview. Br J Nutr. 2000; 84(suppl 1):S3-S10.

- Skinner JD, Bounds W, Carruth BR, Ziegler P. Longitudinal calcium intake is negatively related to children's body fat indexes. J Am Diet Assoc. 2003 Dec;103(12):1626–31.

- Teegarden D, Zemel MB. Dairy product components and weight regulation: symposium overview. J Nutr. 2003;133:243S-244S.

- Teegarden D. Calcium intake and reduction in weight or fat mass. J Nutr. 2003; 133(1):249S-251S. www.jacn.org

- Thoreux K, Schmucker DL. Kefir milk enhances intestinal immunity in young but not old rats. J Nutr. 2001 Mar;131(3):807–12.

- Wang KY, Li SN, Liu CS, Perng DS, Su YC, Wu DC, Jan CM, Lai CH, Wang TN, Wang WM. Effects of ingesting Lactobacillus- and Bifidobacterium-containing yogurt in subjects with colonized Helicobacter pylori. Am J Clin Nutr. 2004 Sep;80(3):737–41.

- Xiao JZ, Kondo S, Takahashi N, Miyaji K, Oshida K, Hiramatsu A, Iwatsuki K, Kokubo S, Hosono A. Effects of milk products fermented by Bifidobacterium longum on blood lipids in rats and healthy adult male volunteers. J Dairy Sci. 2003 Jul;86(7):2452–61.

- Zemel MB, Miller SL. Dietary calcium and dairy modulation of adiposity and obesity risk. Nutr Rev. 2004 Apr;62(4):125–31. Review.

- Zemel MB, Shi H, Zemel PC, DiRienzo D. Calcium and calcium-rich dairy products reduce body fat. FASEB J. 1999 12:LB211(abs.).

- Zemel MB, Thompson W, Milstead A, Morris K, Campbell P. Calcium and dairy acceleration of weight and fat loss during energy restriction in obese adults. Obes Res. 2004 Apr;12(4):582–90.

- Zemel MB. Nutritional and endocrine modulation of intracellular calcium: implications in obesity, insulin resistance and hypertension. Mol Cell Biochem. 1998 Nov;188(1–2):129–36. Review.

- Zemel MB. Regulation of adiposity and obesity risk by dietary calcium: mechanisms and implications. J Am Coll Nutr. 2002 Apr;21(2):146S-151S. Review.

- Zemel MB. Role of calcium and dairy products in energy partitioning and weight management. Am J Clin Nutr. 2004 May;79(5):907S-912S. Review.

#9: Whole Grains

- Adom KK, Liu RH. Antioxidant activity of grains. J Agric Food Chem. 2002 Oct 9;50(21):6182-7.

- Adom KK, Sorrells ME, Liu RH. Phytochemical profiles and antioxidant activity of wheat varieties. J Agric Food Chem. 2003 Dec 17;51(26):7825-34.

- Adom KK, Sorrells ME, Liu RH. Phytochemicals and antioxidant activity of milled fractions of different wheat varieties. J Agric Food Chem. 2005 Mar 23;53(6):2297-306.

- Bazzano LA, He J, Ogden LG, Loria CM, Whelton PK. Dietary fiber intake and reduced risk of coronary heart disease in US men and women: the National Health and Nutrition Examination Survey I Epidemiologic Follow-up Study. Arch Intern Med. 2003 Sep 8;163(16):1897-904.

- Bhathena SJ, Velasquez MT. Beneficial role of dietary phytoestrogens in obesity and diabetes. Am J Clin Nutr. 2002 Dec;76(6):1191-201. Review.

- Chen CY, Milbury PE, Kwak HK, Collins FW, Samuel P, Blumberg JB. Avenanthramides phenolic acids from oats are bioavailable and act synergistically with vitamin C to enhance hamster and human LDL resistance to oxidation. J Nutr. 2004 Jun;134(6):1459-66.

- Delaney B, Nicolosi RJ, Wilson TA et al. Beta-glucan fractions from barley and oats are similarly antiatherogenic in hypercholesterolemic Syrian golden hamsters. J Nutr. 2003 Feb;133(2):468-75.

- Fasano A, Berti I, Gerarduzzi T, Not T, Colletti RB, Drago S, Elitsur Y, Green PH, Guandalini S, Hill ID, Pietzak M, Ventura A, Thorpe M, Kryszak D, Fornaroli F, Wasserman SS, Murray JA, Horvath K. Prevalence of celiac disease in at-risk and not-at-risk groups in the United States: a large multicenter study. Arch Intern Med. 2003 Feb 10;163(3):286-92.

- Fasano A, Catassi C. Coeliac disease in children. Best Pract Res Clin Gastroenterol. 2005 Jun;19(3):467–78.
- Foster-Powell K, Holt SH, Brand-Miller JC. International table of glycemic index and glycemic load values: 2002. Am J Clin Nutr. 2002 Jul;76(1):5–56.
- Jacobs DR Jr, Pereira MA, Stumpf K, Pins JJ, Adlercreutz H. Whole grain food intake elevates serum enterolactone. Br J Nutr. 2002 Aug;88(2):111–6.
- Jayagopal V, Albertazzi P, Kilpatrick ES, Howarth EM, Jennings PE, Hepburn DA, Atkin SL. Beneficial effects of soy phytoestrogen intake in postmenopausal women with type 2 diabetes. Diabetes Care. 2002 Oct;25(10):1709–14.
- Jenkins AL, Jenkins DJ, Zdravkovic U, Wursch P, Vuksan V. Depression of the glycemic index by high levels of beta-glucan fiber in two functional foods tested in type 2 diabetes. Eur J Clin Nutr. 2002 Jul;56(7):622–8.
- Koh-Banerjee P, Franz M, Sampson L, Liu S, Jacobs DR Jr, Spiegelman D, Willett W, Rimm E. Changes in whole-grain, bran, and cereal fiber consumption in relation to 8-y weight gain among men. Am J Clin Nutr. 2004 Nov;80(5):1237–45.
- Liese AD, Roach AK, Sparks KC, Marquart L, D'Agostino RB Jr, Mayer-Davis EJ. Whole-grain intake and insulin sensitivity: the Insulin Resistance Atherosclerosis Study. Am J Clin Nutr. 2003 Nov;78(5):965–71.
- Liu L, Zubik L, Collins FW, Marko M, Meydani M. The antiatherogenic potential of oat phenolic compounds. Atherosclerosis. 2004 Jul;175(1):39–49.
- Liu S, Willett WC, Manson JE, Hu FB, Rosner B, Colditz G. Relation between changes in intakes of dietary fiber and grain products and changes in weight and development of obesity among middle-aged women. Am J Clin Nutr. 2003 Nov;78(5):920–7.
- Pick ME, Hawrysh ZJ, Gee MI, Toth E, Garg ML, Hardin RT. Oat bran concentrate bread products improve long-term control of diabetes: a pilot study. J Am Diet Assoc. 1996 Dec;96(12):1254–61.
- Storsrud S, Olsson M, Arvidsson Lenner R, Nilsson LA, Nilsson O, Kilander A. Adult coeliac patients do tolerate large amounts of oats. Eur J Clin Nutr. 2003 Jan;57(1):163–9.
- The Glycemic Index. School of Molecular and Microbial Biosciences, University of Sydney, NSW, Australia. Accessed online May 26, 2005 at www.glycemicindex.com

#10: Vibrant Vegetables

◆ Arts IC, Hollman PC. Polyphenols and disease risk in epidemiologic studies. Am J Clin Nutr. 2005 Jan;81(1 Suppl):317S-325S. Review.

◆ Bianchini F, Vainio H. Isothiocyanates in cancer prevention. Drug Metab Rev. 2004 Oct;36(3–4):655–67. Review.

◆ Brandi G, Schiavano GF, Zaffaroni N, De Marco C, Paiardini M, Cervasi B, Magnani M. Mechanisms of action and antiproliferative properties of brassica oleracea juice in human breast cancer cell lines. J Nutr. 2005 Jun;135(6):1503–9.

◆ Campbell JK, Canene-Adams K, Lindshield BL, Boileau TW, Clinton SK, Erdman JW Jr. Tomato phytochemicals and prostate cancer risk. J Nutr. 2004 Dec;134(12 Suppl):3486S-3492S. Review.

◆ Fahey JW, Zhang Y, Talalay P. Broccoli sprouts: an exceptionally rich source of inducers of enzymes that protect against chemical carcinogens. Proc Natl Acad Sci U S A. 1997 Sep 16;94(19):10367–72.

◆ Frances, FJ. Pigments and other colorants. In: Food Chemistry (2nd edition) Fennema, OR (ed). New York, NY: Marcel Dekker, Inc, 1985.

◆ Flagg EW, Coates RJ, Greenberg RS. Epidemiologic studies of antioxidants and cancer in humans. J Am Coll Nutr. 1995;14:419–427.

◆ Giovannucci E. Tomatoes, tomato-based products, lycopene, and cancer: review of the epidemiologic literature. J Natl Cancer Inst. 1999;91:317–31.

◆ Goldberg J, Flowerdew G, Smith E, et al. Factors associated with age-related macular degeneration. An analysis of data from the first National Health and Nutrition Examination Survey. Am J Epidemiol. 1988;128:700–710.

◆ Hackett, AM. In: Plant Flavonoids in Biology and Medicine: Biochemical Pharmacological and Structure Activity Relationships. Cody V, Middleton EJ, Harborne JB, (eds) New York: Liss, 1986, 177–94.

◆ Han B, Jaurequi J, Tang BW, Nimni ME. Proanthocyanidin: a natural crosslinking reagent for stabilizing collagen matrices. J Biomed Mater Res. 2003 Apr 1;65A(1):118–24.

◆ Hensrud DD. Diet and obesity. Curr Opin Gastroenterol. 2004 Mar;20(2):119–24.

◆ Holick CN, Michaud DS, Stolzenberg-Solomon R, Mayne ST, Pietinen P, Taylor PR, Virtamo J, Albanes D. Dietary carotenoids, serum beta-carotene, and retinol and risk of lung cancer in the alpha-tocopherol, beta-carotene cohort study. Am J Epidemiol. 2002 Sep 15;156(6):536–47.

♦ Hou DX, Kai K, Li JJ, Lin S, Terahara N, Wakamatsu M, Fujii M, Young MR, Colburn N. Anthocyanidins inhibit activator protein 1 activity and cell transformation: structure-activity relationship and molecular mechanisms. Carcinogenesis. 2004 Jan;25(1):29–36. Epub 2003 Sep 26.

♦ Hou DX. Potential mechanisms of cancer chemoprevention by anthocyanins. Curr Mol Med. 2003 Mar;3(2):149–59. Review.

♦ Ito Y, Gajalakshmi KC, Sasaki R, Suzuki K, Shanta V. A study on serum carotenoid levels in breast cancer patients of Indian women in Chennai (Madras), India. J Epidemiol. 1999 Nov;9(5):306–14.

♦ Kant AK, Graubard BI. Energy density of diets reported by American adults: association with food group intake, nutrient intake, and body weight. Int J Obes Relat Metab Disord. 2005 May 17; [Epub ahead of print].

♦ Keck AS, Finley JW. Cruciferous vegetables: cancer protective mechanisms of glucosinolate hydrolysis products and selenium. Integr Cancer Ther. 2004 Mar;3(1):5–12.

♦ Krinsky NI, Landrum JT, Bone RA. Biologic mechanisms of the protective role of lutein and zeaxanthin in the eye. Annu Rev Nutr. 2003;23:171–201. Epub 2003 Feb 27. Review.

♦ Krinsky NI. Micronutrients and their influence on mutagenicity and malignant transformation. Ann N Y Acad Sci. 1993 May 28;686:229–42. Review.

♦ Kris-Etherton PM, Hecker KD, Bonanome A, Coval SM, Binkoski AE, Hilpert KF, Griel AE, Etherton TD. Bioactive compounds in foods: their role in the prevention of cardiovascular disease and cancer. Am J Med. 2002 Dec 30;113 Suppl 9B:71S-88S. Review.

♦ La Vecchia C, Tavani A. Fruit and vegetables, and human cancer. Eur J Cancer Prev. 1998 Feb;7(1):3–8. Review.

♦ Lamson DW, Brignall MS. Antioxidants and cancer, part 3: quercetin. Altern Med Rev. 2000 Jun;5(3):196–208. Review.

♦ Lee EH, Faulhaber D, Hanson KM, Ding W, Peters S, Kodali S, Granstein RD. Dietary lutein reduces ultraviolet radiation-induced inflammation and immunosuppression. J Invest Dermatol. 2004 Feb;122(2):510–7.

◆ Liu RH. Potential synergy of phytochemicals in cancer prevention: mechanism of action. J Nutr. 2004 Dec;134(12 Suppl):3479S-3485S. Review.

◆ Mazza G, Miniati E. Small fruits. In: Anthocyanins in Fruits, Vegetables, and Grains. Boca Raton, FL: CRC Press, 1993, 85–130.

◆ McBride J. High-ORAC foods may slow aging. USDA Agricultural Research Service website. www.ars.usda.gov/is/pr/1999/990208.htm

◆ Micozzi MS, Beecher GR, Taylor PR, Khachik F. Carotenoid analyses of selected raw and cooked foods associated with a lower risk for cancer. J Natl Cancer Inst. 1990 Feb 21;82(4):282–5. Erratum in: J Natl Cancer Inst 1990 Apr 18;82(8):715.

◆ Moeller SM, Jacques PF, Blumberg JB. The potential role of dietary xantho-phylls in cataract and age-related macular degeneration. J Am Coll Nutr. 2000 Oct;19(5 Suppl):522S-527S. Review.

◆ Robert AM, Tixier JM, Robert L, Legeais JM, Renard G. Effect of pro-cyanidolic oligomers on the permeability of the blood-brain barrier. Pathol Biol (Paris). 2001 May;49(4):298–304.

◆ Rock CL, Saxe GA, Ruffin MT IV, et al. Carotenoids, vitamin A, and estrogen receptor status in breast cancer. Nutr Cancer. 1996;25:281–296.

◆ Rolls BJ, Ello-Martin JA, Tohill BC. What can intervention studies tell us about the relationship between fruit and vegetable consumption and weight manage-ment? Nutr Rev. 2004 Jan;62(1):1–17. Review.

◆ Scalbert A, Johnson IT, Saltmarsh M. Polyphenols: antioxidants and beyond. Am J Clin Nutr. 2005 Jan;81(1 Suppl):215S-217S. Review.

◆ Schmidt K. Antioxidant vitamins and beta-carotene: effects on immunocompe-tence. Am J Clin Nutr. 1991 Jan;53(1 Suppl):383S-385S.

◆ Seddon JM, Ajani UA, Sperduto RD, et al. Dietary carotenoids, vitamins A, C, and E, and advanced age-related macular degeneration. Eye Disease Case-Control Study Group. JAMA. 1994;272:1413–1420.

◆ Seeram NP, Zhang Y, Nair MG. Inhibition of proliferation of human cancer cells and cyclooxygenase enzymes by anthocyanidins and catechins. Nutr Can-cer. 2003;46(1):101–6.

◆ Shapiro TA, Fahey JW, Wade KL, Stephenson KK, Talalay P. Chemoprotective glucosinolates and isothiocyanates of broccoli sprouts: metabolism and excre-tion in humans. Cancer Epidemiol Biomarkers Prev. 2001 May;10(5):501–8.

◆ Slavin JL. Dietary fiber and body weight. Nutrition. 2005 Mar;21(3):411–8.

◆ Spencer JP, Schroeter H, Rechner AR, Rice-Evans C. Bioavailability of flavan-3-ols and procyanidins: gastrointestinal tract influences and their relevance to bioactive forms in vivo. Antioxid Redox Signal. 2001 Dec;3(6):1023–39. Review.

◆ Steinmetz KA, Potter JD. Vegetables, fruit, and cancer prevention: a review. J Am Diet Assoc. 1996 Oct;96(10):1027–39. Review.

◆ Tan WF, Lin LP, Li MH, Zhang YX, Tong YG, Xiao D, Ding J. Quercetin, a dietary-derived flavonoid, possesses antiangiogenic potential. Eur J Pharmacol. 2003 Jan 17;459(2–3):255–62.

◆ The Polyphenol Flavonoids Content and Anti-Oxidant Activities of Various Juices: A Comparative Study. The Lipid Research Laboratory, Technion Faculty of Medicine, The Rappaport Family Institute for Research in the Medical Sciences and Rambam Medical Center, Haifa, Israel.

◆ Toniolo P, Van Kappel AL, Akhmedkhanov A, Ferrari P, Kato I, Shore RE, Riboli E. Serum carotenoids and breast cancer. Am J Epidemiol. 2001 Jun 15;153(12):1142–7.

◆ Van Doorn HE, van der Kruk GC, van Holst GJ. Large scale determination of glucosinolates in brussels sprouts samples after degradation of endogenous glucose. J Agric Food Chem. 1999 Mar;47(3):1029–34.

◆ Vita JA. Polyphenols and cardiovascular disease: effects on endothelial and platelet function. Am J Clin Nutr. 2005 Jan;81(1 Suppl):292S–297S. Review.

◆ Vitale S, West S, Hallfrish J, et al. Plasma antioxidants and risk of cortical and nuclear cataract. Epidemiology. 1993;4:195–203.

◆ Wang H, Cao G, Prior RL. Total antioxidant capacity of fruits. Journal of Agricultural and Food Chemistry. 1996;44(3):701–705.

◆ Yao LH, Jiang YM, Shi J, Tomas-Barberan FA, Datta N, Singanusong R, Chen SS. Flavonoids in food and their health benefits. Plant Foods Hum Nutr. 2004 Summer;59(3):113–22. Review.

◆ Zhang LX et al. Carotenoids enhance hap junctional communication and inhibit lipid peroxidation in C3H/10T1/2 cells: Relationship to their cancer chemopreventive action. Carcinogenesis. 12:2109–2114 (1991).

◆ Ziegler RG. Vegetables, fruits, and carotenoids and the risk of cancer. Am J Clin Nutr. 1991 Jan;53(1 Suppl):251S-259S. Review.

Omega-3 EFAs

- Browning LM. N-3 polyunsaturated fatty acids, inflammation and obesity-related disease. Proc Nutr Soc. 2003 May;62(2):447–53. Review.

- Clarke SD, Thuillier P, Baillie RA, Sha X. Peroxisome proliferator-activated receptors: a family of lipid-activated transcription factors. Am J Clin Nutr. 1999 Oct;70(4):566–71. Biochimie. 1998;79:95–99. Review.

- Clarke SD. Polyunsaturated fatty acid regulation of gene transcription: a mechanism to improve energy balance and insulin resistance. Br J Nutr. 2000 Mar;83 Suppl 1:S59–66. Review.

- Clarke SD. Polyunsaturated fatty acid regulation of gene transcription: a mechanism to improve energy balance and insulin resistance. Br J Nutr. 2000 Mar;83 Suppl 1:S59–66. Review.

- Delarue J, LeFoll C, Corporeau C, Lucas D. N-3 long chain polyunsaturated fatty acids: a nutritional tool to prevent insulin resistance associated to type 2 diabetes and obesity? Reprod Nutr Dev. 2004 May-Jun;44(3):289–99. Review.

- Duplus E, Glorian M, Forest C. Fatty acid regulation of gene transcription. J Biol Chem. 2000 Oct 6;275(40):30749–52. Review.

- Field FJ, Born E, Murthy S, Mathur SN. Polyunsaturated fatty acids decrease the expression of sterol regulatory element-binding protein-1 in CaCo-2 cells: effect on fatty acid synthesis and triacylglycerol transport. Biochem J. 2002 Dec 15; 368(Pt 3):855–64.

- Garvey WT. The role of uncoupling protein 3 in human physiology. J Clin Invest. 2003 Feb;111(4):438–41.

- Jump DB, Clarke SD. Regulation of gene expression by dietary fat. Annu Rev Nutr. 1999;19:63–90. Review.

- Kuriki K, Nagaya T, Tokudome Y, Imaeda N, Fujiwara N, Sato J, Goto C, Ikeda M, Maki S, Tajima K, Tokudome S. Plasma concentrations of (n-3) highly unsaturated fatty acids are good biomarkers of relative dietary fatty acid intakes: a cross-sectional study. J Nutr. 2003 Nov;133(11):3643–50.

- Li H, Ruan XZ, Powis SH, Fernando R, Mon WY, Wheeler DC, Moorhead JF, Varghese Z. EPA and DHA reduce LPS-induced inflammation responses in

HK-2 cells: evidence for a PPAR-gamma-dependent mechanism. Kidney Int. 2005 Mar;67(3):867–74.

◆ Lovejoy JC. The influence of dietary fat on insulin resistance. Curr Diab Rep. 2002 Oct;2(5):435–40. Review.

◆ Manco M, Calvani M, Mingrone G. Effects of dietary fatty acids on insulin sensitivity and secretion. Diabetes Obes Metab. 2004 Nov;6(6):402–13. Review.

◆ Massiera F, Saint-Marc P, Seydoux J, Murata T, Kobayashi T, Narumiya S, Guesnet P, Amri EZ, Negrel R, Ailhaud G. Arachidonic acid and prostacyclin signaling promote adipose tissue development: a human health concern? J Lipid Res. 2003 Feb;44(2):271–9. Epub 2002 Nov 04.

◆ Mishra A, Chaudhary A, Sethi S. Oxidized omega-3 fatty acids inhibit NF-kappaB activation via a PPARalpha-dependent pathway. Arterioscler Thromb Vasc Biol. 2004 Sep;24(9):1621–7. Epub 2004 Jul 1.

◆ Mori TA, Bao DQ, Burke V, Puddey IB, Watts GF, Beilin LJ. Dietary fish as a major component of a weight-loss diet: effect on serum lipids, glucose, and insulin metabolism in overweight hypertensive subjects. Am J Clin Nutr. 1999 Nov;70(5):817–25.

◆ Mori TA, Burke V, Puddey IB, Shaw JE, Beilin LJ. Effect of fish diets and weight loss on serum leptin concentration in overweight, treated-hypertensive subjects. J Hypertens. 2004 Oct;22(10):1983–90.

◆ Oudart H, Groscolas R, Calgari C, Nibbelink M, Leray C, Le Maho Y, Malan A. Brown fat thermogenesis in rats fed high-fat diets enriched with n-3 polyunsaturated fatty acids. Int J Obes Relat Metab Disord. 1997 Nov;21(11):955–62.

◆ Pischon T, Hankinson SE, Hotamisligil GS, Rifai N, Willett WC, Rimm EB. Habitual dietary intake of n-3 and n-6 fatty acids in relation to inflammatory markers among US men and women. Circulation. 2003 Jul 15;108(2):155–60. Epub 2003 Jun 23.

◆ Power GW, Newsholme EA. Dietary fatty acids influence the activity and metabolic control of mitochondrial carnitine palmitoyltransferase I in rat heart and skeletal muscle. J Nutr. 1997 Nov;127(11):2142–50.

◆ Rivellese AA, Lilli S. Quality of dietary fatty acids, insulin sensitivity and type 2 diabetes. Biomed Pharmacother. 2003 Mar;57(2):84–7. Review.

◆ Sessler AM, Ntambi JM. Polyunsaturated fatty acid regulation of gene expression. J Nutr. 1998 Jun;128(6):923–6. Review.

♦ Simopoulos AP. Omega-3 fatty acids in inflammation and autoimmune diseases. J Am Coll Nutr. 2002 Dec;21(6):495–505.

♦ Sulzle A, Hirche F, Eder K. Thermally oxidized dietary fat upregulates the expression of target genes of PPAR alpha in rat liver. J Nutr. 2004 Jun;134(6):1375–83.

♦ Ukropec J, Reseland JE, Gasperikova D, Demcakova E, Madsen L, Berge RK, Rustan AC, Klimes I, Drevon CA, Sebokova E. The hypotriglyceridemic effect of dietary n-3 FA is associated with increased beta-oxidation and reduced leptin expression. Lipids. 2003 Oct;38(10):1023–9.

♦ Vessby B, Unsitupa M, Hermansen K, Riccardi G, Rivellese AA, Tapsell LC, Nalsen C, Berglund L, Louheranta A, Rasmussen BM, Calvert GD, Maffetone A, Pedersen E, Gustafsson IB, Storlien LH; KANWU Study. Substituting dietary saturated for monounsaturated fat impairs insulin sensitivity in healthy men and women: The KANWU Study. Diabetologia. 2001 Mar;44(3):312–9.

♦ Wang YX, Lee CH, Tiep S, Yu RT, Ham J, Kang H, Evans RM. Peroxisome-proliferator-activated receptor delta activates fat metabolism to prevent obesity. Cell. 2003 Apr 18;113(2):159–70.

♦ Yamauchi T, Waki H, Kamon J, Murakami K, Motojima K, Komeda K, Miki H, Kubota N, Terauchi Y, Tsuchida A, Tsuboyama-Kasaoka N, Yamauchi N, Ide T, Hori W, Kato S, Fukayama M, Akanuma Y, Ezaki O, Itai A, Nagai R, Kimura S, Tobe K, Kagechika H, Shudo K, Kadowaki T. Inhibition of RXR and PPARgamma ameliorates diet-induced obesity and type 2 diabetes. J Clin Invest. 2001 Oct;108(7):1001–13.

♦ Zhao Y, Joshi-Barve S, Barve S, Chen LH. Eicosapentaenoic acid prevents LPS-induced TNF-alpha expression by preventing NF-kappaB activation. J Am Coll Nutr. 2004 Feb;23(1):71–8.

Alpha Lipoic Acid

♦ Bierhaus A, et al. Advanced glycation end product-induced activation of NF-kappaB is suppressed by alpha-lipoic acid in cultured endothelial cells. Diabetes. 1997 Sep;46(9):1481–90.

♦ Cakatay U, Telci A, Kayali R, Sivas A, Akcay T. Effect of alpha-lipoic acid supplementation on oxidative protein damage in the streptozotocin-diabetic rat. Res Exp Med (Berl). 2000 Feb;199(4):243–51.

♦ Evans JL, Goldfine ID. Alpha-lipoic acid: a multifunctional antioxidant that improves insulin sensitivity in patients with type 2 diabetes. Diabetes Technol Ther. 2000 Autumn;2(3):401–13. Review.

♦ Fuchs J, Milbradt R. Antioxidant inhibition of skin inflammation induced by reactive oxidants: evaluation of the redox couple dihydrolipoate/lipoate. Skin Pharmacol. 1994;7(5):278–84.

♦ Han D, Handelman G, Marcocci L, Sen CK, Roy S, Kobuchi H, Tritschler HJ, Flohe L, Packer L. Lipoic acid increases de novo synthesis of cellular glutathione by improving cystine utilization. Biofactors. 1997;6(3):321–38.

♦ Kagan VE, Shvedova A, Serbinova E, Khan S, Swanson C, Powell R, Packer L. Dihydrolipoic acid—a universal antioxidant both in the membrane and in the aqueous phase. Reduction of peroxyl, ascorbyl and chromanoxyl radicals. Biochem Pharmacol. 1992 Oct 20;44(8):1637–49.

♦ Kocak G, Aktan F, Canbolat O, Ozogul C, Elbeg S, Yildizoglu-Ari N, Karasu C. Alpha-lipoic acid treatment ameliorates metabolic parameters, blood pressure, vascular reactivity and morphology of vessels already damaged by streptozotocin-diabetes. Diabetes Nutr Metab. 2000 Dec;13(6):308–18.

♦ Kunt T, et al. Alpha-lipoic acid reduces expression of vascular cell adhesion molecule-1 and endothelial adhesion of human monocytes after stimulation with advanced glycation end products. Clin Sci (Lond). 1999 Jan;96(1):75–82.

♦ Linetsky M, James HL, Ortwerth BJ. Spontaneous generation of superoxide anion by human lens proteins and by calf lens proteins ascorbylated in vitro. Exp Eye Res. 1999 Aug;69(2):239–48.

♦ Melhem MF, Craven PA, Derubertis FR. Effects of dietary supplementation of alpha-lipoic acid on early glomerular injury in diabetes mellitus. J Am Soc Nephrol. 2001 Jan;12(1):124–33.

♦ Melhem MF, Craven PA, Liachenko J, DeRubertis FR. Alpha-lipoic acid attenuates hyperglycemia and prevents glomerular mesangial matrix expansion in diabetes. J Am Soc Nephrol. 2002 Jan;13(1):108–16.

♦ Meyer M, Pahl HL, Baeuerle PA. Regulation of the transcription factors NF-kappa B and AP-1 by redox changes. Chem Biol Interact. 1994 Jun;91(2–3):91–100.

♦ Meyer M, Schreck R, Baeuerle PA. H2O2 and antioxidants have opposite effects on activation of NF-kappa B and AP-1 in intact cells: AP-1 as secondary antioxidant-responsive factor. EMBO J. 1993 May;12(5):2005–15.

◆ Ookawara T, Kawamura N, Kitagawa Y, Taniguchi N. Site-specific and random fragmentation of Cu, Zn-superoxide dismutase by glycation reaction. Implication of reactive oxygen species. J Biol Chem. 1992 Sep 15;267(26):18505–10.

◆ Packer L, Kraemer K, Rimbach G. Molecular aspects of lipoic acid in the prevention of diabetes complications. Nutrition. 2001 Oct;17(10):888–95. Review.

◆ Packer L, Roy S, Sen CK. A-lipoic acid: a metabolic antioxidant and potential redox modulator of transcription. Advances in Pharmacology. 1996; 38: 79–101.

◆ Packer L, Witt EH, Tritschler HJ. Alpha-lipoic acid as a biological antioxidant. Free Radic Biol Med. 1995 Aug;19(2):227–50. Review.

◆ Perricone N, Nagy, K, Horvath F, Dajko G, Uray I, Zs-Nagy I. Alpha lipoic acid (ALA) protects proteins against the hydroxyl free radical-induced alterations: rationale for its geriatric application. Arch Gerontol Geriatr. 1999 Jul–Aug; 29(1): 45–56.

◆ Perricone NV. Topical 5% alpha lipoic acid cream in the treatment of cutaneous rhytids. Aesthetic Surg J. 2000 May–Jun; 20(3).

◆ Podda M, Rallis M, Traber MG, Packer L, Maibach HI. Kinetic study of cutaneous and subcutaneous distribution following topical application of [7,8–14C]rac-alpha-lipoic acid onto hairless mice. Biochem Pharmacol. 1996 Aug 23;52(4):627–33.

◆ Podda M, Tritschler HJ, Ulrich H, Packer L. Alpha-lipoic acid supplementation prevents symptoms of vitamin E deficiency. Biochem Biophys Res Commun. 1994 Oct 14;204(1):98–104.

◆ Podda M, Zollner TM, Grundmann-Kollmann M, Thiele JJ, Packer L, Kaufmann R. Activity of alpha-lipoic acid in the protection against oxidative stress in skin. Curr Probl Dermatol. 2001;29:43–51.

◆ Roy S, Sen CK, Tritschler HJ, Packer L. Modulation of cellular reducing equivalent homeostasis by alpha-lipoic acid. Mechanisms and implications for diabetes and ischemic injury. Biochem Pharmacol. 1997 Feb 7;53(3):393–9.

◆ Saliou C, Kitazawa M, McLaughlin L, Yang JP, Lodge JK, Tetsuka T, Iwasaki K, Cillard J, Okamoto T, Packer L. Antioxidants modulate acute solar ultraviolet

radiation-induced NF-kappa-B activation in a human keratinocyte cell line. Free
Radic Biol Med. 1999 Jan;26(1–2):174–83.

- Sen CK, Packer L. Antioxidant and redox regulation of gene transcription.
  FASEB J. 1996; 10: 709–720.

- Suzuki YJ, Aggarwal BB, Packer L. Alpha-lipoic acid is a potent inhibitor of
  NF-kappa B activation in human T cells. Biochem Biophys Res Commun.
  1992 Dec 30;189(3):1709–15.

- Suzuki YJ, Mizuno M, Tritschler HJ, Packer L. Redox regulation of NF-
  kappa B DNA binding activity by dihydrolipoate. Biochem Mol Biol Int.
  1995 Jun;36(2):241–6.

- Suzuki YJ, Tsuchiya M, Packer L. Lipoate prevents glucose-induced protein
  modifications. Free Radic Res Commun. 1992;17(3):211–7.

- Ziegler D, Reljanovic M, Mehnert H, Gries FA. Alpha-lipoic acid in the treatment of diabetic polyneuropathy in Germany: current evidence from clinical trials. Exp Clin Endocrinol Diabetes. 1999;107(7):421–30. Review.

Astaxanthin

- Ben-Dor A, Steiner M, Gheber L, Danilenko M, Dubi N, Linnewiel K, Zick A,
  Sharoni Y, Levy J. Carotenoids activate the antioxidant response element transcription system. Mol Cancer Ther. 2005 Jan;4(1):177–86.

- Bennedsen M, Wang X, Willen R, Wadstrom T, Andersen LP. Treatment of H.
  pylori infected mice with antioxidant astaxanthin reduces gastric inflammation,
  bacterial load and modulates cytokine release by splenocytes. Immunol Lett.
  1999 Dec 1;70(3):185–9.

- Guerin M, Huntley ME, Olaizola M. Haematococcus astaxanthin: applications for
  human health and nutrition. Trends Biotechnol. 2003 May;21(5):210–6. Review.

- Kurashige M, Okimasu E, Inoue M, Utsumi K. Inhibition of oxidative injury
  of biological membranes by astaxanthin. Physiol Chem Phys Med NMR.
  1990;22(1):27–38.

- Lauver DA, Lockwood SF, Lucchesi BR. Disodium disuccinate astaxanthin
  (CardaxTM) attenuates complement activation and reduces myocardial injury
  following ischemia/reperfusion. J Pharmacol Exp Ther. 2005 May 4; [Epub
  ahead of print].

- Ohgami K, Shiratori K, Kotake S, Nishida T, Mizuki N, Yazawa K, Ohno S. Effects of astaxanthin on lipopolysaccharide-induced inflammation in vitro and in vivo. Invest Ophthalmol Vis Sci. 2003 Jun;44(6):2694–701.
- Wang X, Willen R, Wadstrom T. Astaxanthin-rich algal meal and vitamin C inhibit Helicobacter pylori infection in BALB/cA mice. Antimicrob Agents Chemother. 2000 Sep;44(9):2452–7.

Carnitine

- [No authors listed]. L-carnitine. Med Lett Drugs Ther. 2004 Nov 22;46(1196):95–6.
- Brandsch C, Eder K. Effect of L-carnitine on weight loss and body composition of rats fed a hypocaloric diet. Ann Nutr Metab. 2002;46(5):205–10.
- Center SA, Harte J, Watrous D, Reynolds A, Watson TD, Markwell PJ, Millington DS, Wood PA, Yeager AE, Erb HN. The clinical and metabolic effects of rapid weight loss in obese pet cats and the influence of supplemental oral L-carnitine. J Vet Intern Med. 2000 Nov-Dec;14(6):598–608.
- He Z-Q, Phone ZS. Body weight reduction in adolescents by a combination of measures including using L-carnitine. Acta Nutrimenta Sinica. 1997;19(2).
- Hongu N, Sachan DS. Carnitine and choline supplementation with exercise alter carnitine profiles, biochemical markers of fat metabolism and serum leptin concentration in healthy women. J Nutr. 2003 Jan;133(1):84–9.
- Lurz R, Fischer R. Aerztezeitschrift fur Naturheilverfahren. 1998; 39(12).
- Muller DM, Seim H, Kiess W, Loster H, Richter T. Effects of oral L-carnitine supplementation on in vivo long-chain fatty acid oxidation in healthy adults. Metabolism. 2002 Nov;51(11):1389–91.
- Saldanha Aoki M, Rodriguez Amaral Almeida AL, Navarro F, Bicudo Pereira Costa-Rosa LF, Pereira Bacurau RF. Carnitine supplementation fails to maximize fat mass loss induced by endurance training in rats. Ann Nutr Metab. 2004;48(2):90–4. Epub 2004 Feb 25.
- Villani RG, Gannon J, Self M, Rich PA. L-carnitine supplementation combined with aerobic training does not promote weight loss in moderately obese women. Int J Sport Nutr Exerc Metab. 2000 Jun;10(2):199–207.
- Wutzke KD, Lorenz H. The effect of l-carnitine on fat oxidation, protein

turnover, and body composition in slightly overweight subjects. Metabolism. 2004 Aug;53(8):1002–6.

Acetyl-L-carnitine

- Ames BN, Liu J. Delaying the mitochondrial decay of aging with acetylcarnitine. Ann N Y Acad Sci. 2004 Nov;1033:108–16. Review.
- Ames BN. Delaying the mitochondrial decay of aging. Ann N Y Acad Sci. 2004 Jun;1019:406–11. Review.
- Beal MF. Bioenergetic approaches for neuroprotection in Parkinson's disease. Ann Neurol. 2003;53 Suppl 3:S39–47; Discussion S47–8. Review.
- Hagen TM, Moreau R, Suh JH, Visioli F. Mitochondrial decay in the aging rat heart: evidence for improvement by dietary supplementation with acetyl-L-carnitine and/or lipoic acid. Ann N Y Acad Sci. 2002 Apr;959:491–507. Review.
- Liu J, Atamna H, Kuratsune H, Ames BN. Delaying brain mitochondrial decay and aging with mitochondrial antioxidants and metabolites. Ann N Y Acad Sci. 2002 Apr;959:133–66. Review.
- Mingrone G. Carnitine in type 2 diabetes. Ann N Y Acad Sci. 2004 Nov; 1033:99–107. Review.
- Shigenaga MK, Hagen TM, Ames BN. Oxidative damage and mitochondrial decay in aging. Proc Natl Acad Sci U S A. 1994 Nov 8;91(23):10771–8. Review.

CLA

- Belury MA, et al., The conjugated linoleic acid (CLA) isomer, t10c12-CLA, is inversely associated with changes in body weight and serum leptin in subjects with type 2 diabetes mellitus. J Nutr. 2003; 133(1): 257s–260s.
- Benito P, Nelson GJ, Kelley DS, Bartolini G, Schmidt PC, Simon V. The effect of conjugated linoleic acid on plasma lipoproteins and tissue fatty acid composition in humans. Lipids. 2001 Mar;36(3):229–36. Erratum in: Lipids 2001 Aug;36(8):857.
- Blankson H, Stakkestad JA, Fagertun H, Thom E, Wadstein J, Gudmundsen O. Conjugated linoleic acid reduces body fat mass in overweight and obese humans. J Nutr. 2000 Dec;130(12):2943–8.

◆ Gaullier JM, Halse J, Hoye K, Kristiansen K, Fagertun H, Vik H, Gudmundsen O. Supplementation with conjugated linoleic acid for 24 months is well tolerated by and reduces body fat mass in healthy, overweight humans. J Nutr. 2005 Apr; 135(4):778–84.

◆ Haugen M, Alexander J. [Can linoleic acids in conjugated CLA products reduce overweight problems?]. Tidsskr Nor Laegeforen. 2004 Dec 2;124(23):3051–4. Review. Norwegian.

◆ Kamphuis MM, Lejeune MP, Saris WH, Westerterp-Plantenga MS. Effect of conjugated linoleic acid supplementation after weight loss on appetite and food intake in overweight subjects. Eur J Clin Nutr. 2003 Oct;57(10):1268–74.

◆ Kamphuis MM, Lejeune MP, Saris WH, Westerterp-Plantenga MS. Effect of conjugated linoleic acid supplementation after weight loss on appetite and food intake in overweight subjects. Eur J Clin Nutr. 2003 Oct;57(10):1268–74.

◆ Kamphuis MM, Lejeune MP, Saris WH, Westerterp-Plantenga MS. The effect of conjugated linoleic acid supplementation after weight loss on body weight re-gain, body composition, and resting metabolic rate in overweight subjects. Int J Obes Relat Metab Disord. 2003 Jul;27(7):840–7.

◆ Malpuech-Brugere C, Verboeket-van de Venne WP, Mensink RP, Arnal MA, Morio B, Brandolini M, Saebo A, Lassel TS, Chardigny JM, Sebedio JL, Beaufrere B. Effects of two conjugated linoleic acid isomers on body fat mass in overweight humans. Obes Res. 2004 Apr;12(4):591–8.

◆ Moloney F, Yeow TP, Mullen A, Nolan JJ, Roche HM. Conjugated linoleic acid supplementation, insulin sensitivity, and lipoprotein metabolism in patients with type 2 diabetes mellitus. Am J Clin Nutr. 2004 Oct;80(4):887–95.

◆ Nagao K et al. The 10trans,12cis isomer of conjugated linoleic acid suppresses the development of hypertension in Otsuka Long-Evans Tokushima fatty rats. Biochem Biophys Res Commun. 2003; 306(1):134–8.

◆ Riserus U, Berglund L, Vessby B. Conjugated linoleic acid (CLA) reduced ab-dominal adipose tissue in obese middle-aged men with signs of the metabolic syndrome: a randomised controlled trial. Int J Obes Relat Metab Disord. 2001 Aug;25(8):1129–35.

◆ Riserus U, Vessby B, Arnlov J, Basu S. Effects of cis-9,trans-11 conjugated linoleic acid supplementation on insulin sensitivity, lipid peroxidation, and proinflamma-tory markers in obese men. Am J Clin Nutr. 2004 Aug;80(2):279–83.

- Smedman A, Vessby B. Conjugated linoleic acid supplementation in humans–metabolic effects. Lipids. 2001;36(8):773–81.
- Thom E, et al. Conjugated linoleic acid reduces body fat in healthy exercising humans. J Int Med Res. 2001;29(5)392–6.
- Whigham LD, O'Shea M, Mohede IC, Walaski HP, Atkinson RL. Safety profile of conjugated linoleic acid in a 12-month trial in obese humans. Food Chem Toxicol. 2004 Oct;42(10):1701–9.
- Zambell KL, Keim NL, Van Loan MD, Gale B, Benito P, Kelley DS, Nelson GJ. Conjugated linoleic acid supplementation in humans: effects on body composition and energy expenditure. Lipids. 2000 Jul;35(7):777–82.

CoQ10

- Beal MF. Mitochondria, oxidative damage, and inflammation in Parkinson's disease. Ann N Y Acad Sci. 2003 Jun;991:120–31. Review.
- Beal MF. Mitochondrial dysfunction and oxidative damage in Alzheimer's and Parkinson's diseases and coenzyme Q10 as a potential treatment. J Bioenerg Biomembr. 2004 Aug;36(4):381–6. Review.
- Chew GT, Watts GF. Coenzyme Q10 and diabetic endotheliopathy: oxidative stress and the "recoupling hypothesis." QJM. 2004 Aug;97(8):537–48. Review.
- Crane FL. Biochemical functions of coenzyme Q10. J Am Coll Nutr. 2001 Dec;20(6):591–8. Review.
- Lamson DW, Plaza SM. Mitochondrial factors in the pathogenesis of diabetes: a hypothesis for treatment. Altern Med Rev. 2002 Apr;7(2):94–111. Review.
- Lenaz G, D'Aurelio M, Merlo Pich M, Genova ML, Ventura B, Bovina C, Formiggini G, Parenti Castelli G. Mitochondrial bioenergetics in aging. Biochim Biophys Acta. 2000 Aug 15;1459(2–3):397–404. Review.
- Steele PE, Tang PH, DeGrauw AJ, Miles MV. Clinical laboratory monitoring of coenzyme Q10 use in neurologic and muscular diseases. Am J Clin Pathol. 2004 Jun;121 Suppl:S113–20. Review.

Chromium

- Amato P, Morales AJ, Yen SS. Effects of chromium picolinate supplementation on insulin sensitivity, serum lipids, and body composition in healthy, nonobese, older men and women. J Gerontol A Biol Sci Med Sci. 2000 May;55(5): M260–3.

◆ Anderson RA. Effects of chromium on body composition and weight loss. Nutr Rev. 1998;56:266–70.

◆ Bahadori B, Wallner S, Schneider H, Wascher TC, Toplak H. [Effect of chromium yeast and chromium picolinate on body composition of obese, non-diabetic patients during and after a formula diet]. Acta Med Austriaca. 1997;24(5):185–7. German.

◆ Campbell WW, Joseph LJ, Anderson RA, Davey SL, Hinton J, Evans WJ. Effects of resistive training and chromium picolinate on body composition and skeletal muscle size in older women. Int J Sport Nutr Exerc Metab. 2002 Jun;12(2):125–35.

◆ Campbell WW, Joseph LJ, Davey SL, Cyr-Campbell D, Anderson RA, Evans WJ. Effects of resistance training and chromium picolinate on body composition and skeletal muscle in older men. J Appl Physiol. 1999 Jan;86(1):29–39.

◆ Clancy SP, Clarkson PM, DeCheke ME, Nosaka K, Freedson PS, Cunningham JJ, Valentine B. Effects of chromium picolinate supplementation on body composition, strength, and urinary chromium loss in football players. Int J Sport Nutr. 1994 Jun;4(2):142–53.

◆ Grant KE, Chandler RM, Castle AL, Ivy JL. Chromium and exercise training: effect on obese women. Med Sci Sports Exerc. 1997 Aug;29(8):992–8.

◆ Kaats GR, Blum K, Fisher JA, Adelman JA. Effects of chromium picolinate supplementation on body composition: a randomized, double-masked, placebo-controlled study. Curr Ther Res. 1996;57:747–56.

◆ Kaats GR, Blum K, Pullin D, et al. A randomized, double-masked, placebo-controlled study of the effects of chromium picolinate supplementation on body composition: a replication and extension of a previous study. Curr Ther Res. 1998;59:379–88.

◆ Livolsi JM, Adams GM, Laguna PL. The effect of chromium picolinate on muscular strength and body composition in women athletes. J Strength Cond Res. 2001 May;15(2):161–6.

◆ Pittler MH, Stevinson C, Ernst E. Chromium picolinate for reducing body weight: meta-analysis of randomized trials. Int J Obes Relat Metab Disord. 2003 Apr;27(4):522–9

- Trent LK, Thieding-Cancel D. Effects of chromium picolinate on body composition. J Sports Med Phys Fitness. 1995 Dec;35(4):273–80.

- Vincent JB. The potential value and toxicity of chromium picolinate as a nutritional supplement, weight loss agent and muscle development agent. Sports Med. 2003;33(3):213–30. Review.

- Volpe SL, Huang HW, Larpadisorn K, Lesser II. Effect of chromium supplementation and exercise on body composition, resting metabolic rate and selected biochemical parameters in moderately obese women following an exercise program. J Am Coll Nutr. 2001 Aug;20(4):293–306.

- Walker LS, Bemben MG, Bemben DA, Knehans AW. Chromium picolinate effects on body composition and muscular performance in wrestlers. Med Sci Sports Exerc. 1998 Dec;30(12):1730–7.

GLA

- Cameron NE, Cotter MA, Horrobin DH, et al. Effects of alpha-lipoic acid on neurovascular function in diabetic rats: Interaction with essential fatty acids. Diabetologia. 1998;41:390–399.

- Garcia CM, Carter J, Chou A. Gamma linolenic acid causes weight loss and lower blood pressure in overweight patients with family history of obesity. Swed J Biol Med. 1986;4:8–11.

- Hounsom L, Horrobin DF, Tritschler H, et al. A lipoic acid-gamma linolenic acid conjugate is effective against multiple indices of experimental diabetic neuropathy. Diabetologia. 1998;41:839–843.

- Jamal GA, Carmichael H. The effect of gamma-linolenic acid on human diabetic peripheral neuropathy: a double-blind placebo-controlled trial. Diabet Med. 1990;7:319–323.

- Keen H, Payan J, Allawi J, et al. Treatment of diabetic neuropathy with gamma-linolenic acid. The Gamma-Linolenic Acid Multicenter Trial Group. Diabetes Care. 1993;16:8–15.

- Leventhal LJ, Boyce EG, Zurier RB. Treatment of rheumatoid arthritis with gammalinolenic acid.

- Zurier RB, Rossetti RG, Jacobson EW, et al. gamma-Linolenic acid treatment of rheumatoid arthritis. A randomized, placebo-controlled trial. Arthritis Rheum. 1996;39:1808–1817.

Glutamine

- Castell L. Glutamine supplementation in vitro and in vivo, in exercise and in immunodepression. Sports Med. 2003;33(5):323–45. Review.
- Clark RH, Feleke G, Din M, et al. Nutritional treatment for acquired immunodeficiency virus-associated wasting using beta-hydroxy beta-methylbutyrate, glutamine, and arginine: a randomized, double-blind, placebo-controlled study. J Parenter Enteral Nutr. 2000;24:133–139.
- Curi R, Lagranha CJ, Doi SQ, Sellitti DF, Procopio J, Pithon-Curi TC, Corless M, Newsholme P. Molecular mechanisms of glutamine action. J Cell Physiol. 2005 Aug;204(2):392–401.
- Grimble RF. Nutritional modulation of immune function. Proc Nutr Soc. 2001 Aug;60(3):389–97. Review.
- Opara EC, Petro A, Tevrizian A, Feinglos MN, Surwit RS. L-glutamine supplementation of a high fat diet reduces body weight and attenuates hyperglycemia and hyperinsulinemia in C57BL/6J mice. J Nutr. 1996 Jan;126(1):273–9.
- Rutten EP, Engelen MP, Schols AM, Deutz NE. Skeletal muscle glutamate metabolism in health and disease: state of the art. Curr Opin Clin Nutr Metab Care. 2005 Jan;8(1):41–51. Review.
- Shabert JK, Winslow C, Lacey JM, et al. Glutamine-antioxidant supplementation increases body cell mass in AIDS patients with weight loss: a randomized, double-blind controlled trial. Nutrition. 1999;15:860–864.

Maitake SX Fraction

- Manohar V, Talpur NA, Echard BW, Lieberman S, Preuss HG. Effects of a water-soluble extract of Maitake mushroom on circulating glucose/insulin concentrations in KK mice. Diabetes Obes Metab. 2002 Jan;4(1):43–8.
- Talpur N, Echard B, Dadgar A, Aggarwal S, Zhuang C, Bagchi D, Preuss HG. Effects of Maitake mushroom fractions on blood pressure of Zucker fatty rats. Res Commun Mol Pathol Pharmacol. 2002;112(1–4):68–82.

- Talpur N, Echard BW, Yasmin T, Bagchi D, Preuss HG. Effects of niacin-bound chromium, Maitake mushroom fraction SX and (-)-hydroxycitric acid on the metabolic syndrome in aged diabetic Zucker fatty rats. Mol Cell Biochem. 2003 Oct;252(1–2):369–77.

- Talpur NA, Echard BW, Fan AY, Jaffari O, Bagchi D, Preuss HG. Antihypertensive and metabolic effects of whole Maitake mushroom powder and its fractions in two rat strains. Mol Cell Biochem. 2002 Aug;237(1–2):129–36.

- Wasser SP. Medicinal mushrooms as a source of antitumor and immunomodulating polysaccharides. Appl Microbiol Biotechnol. 2002 Nov;60(3):258–74. Epub 2002 Sep 10. Review.

DMAE

- Alkadhi KA. Endplate channel actions of a hemicholinium-3 analog, DMAE. Naunyn Schmiedebergs Arch Pharmacol. 1986 Mar;332(3):230–5.

- Alvaro D, Cantafora A, Gandin C, Masella R, Santini MT, Angelico M. Selective hepatic enrichment of polyunsaturated phosphatidylcholines after intravenous administration of dimethylethanolamine in the rat. Biochim Biophys Acta. 1989 Nov 6;1006(1):116–20.

- Cole AC, Gisoldi EM, Grossman RM. Clinical and consumer evaluations of improved facial appearance after 1 month use of topical dimethylaminoethanol. Poster Presentation, American Academy of Dermatology, Feb. 22–26, 2002, New Orleans, USA.

- Grossman RM, Gisoldi EM, Cole AC. Long term safety and efficacy evaluation of a new skin firming technology: dimethylaminoethanol. Poster Presentation, American Academy of Dermatology, Feb. 22–26, 2002, New Orleans, Louisiana, USA.

- Grossman RM. The role of dimethylaminoethanol in cosmetic dermatology. Skillman, NJ: Johnson and Johnson Consumer Products Worldwide.

- Nagy I, Floyd RA. Electron spin resonance spectroscopic demonstration of the hydroxyl free radical scavenger properties of dimethylaminoethanol in spin trapping experiments confirming the molecular basis for the biological effects of centrophenoxine. Arch Gerontol Geriatr. 1984 Dec;3(4):297–310.

- Nagy I, Nagy K. On the role of cross-linking of cellular proteins in aging. Mech Aging Dev. 1980 Sep-Oct;14(1–2):245–51.

- Semsei I, Zs-Nagy I. Superoxide radical scavenging ability of centrophenoxine and its salt dependence in vitro. J Free Radic Biol Med. 1985;1(5–6):403–8.
- Yu MJ, et al. Phenothiazines as lipid peroxidation inhibitors and cytoprotective agents. J Med Chem. 1992 Feb 21;35(4):716–24.
- Zs-Nagy I, Semsei I. Centrophenoxine increases the rates of total and mRNA synthesis in the brain cortex of old rats: an explanation of its action in terms of the membrane hypothesis of aging. Exp Gerontol. 1984;19(3):171–8.
- Zs-Nagy I. On the role of intracellular physicochemistry in quantitative gene expression during aging and the effect of centrophenoxine. A review. Arch Gerontol Geriatr. 1989 Nov-Dec;9(3):215–29. Review.

CHAPTER 7: STEP THREE: THE ANTI-INFLAMMATORY LIFESTYLE

- Berk LS, Tan SA, Fry WF, Napier BJ, Lee JW, Hubbard RW, Lewis JE, Eby WC. Neuroendocrine and stress hormone changes during mirthful laughter. Am J Med Sci. 1989 Dec;298(6):390–6.
- Bjorntorp P. Do stress reactions cause abdominal obesity and comorbidities? Obes Rev. 2001 May;2(2):73–86.
- Dallman MF, la Fleur SE, Pecoraro NC, Gomez F, Houshyar H, Akana SF. Mini-review: glucocorticoids–food intake, abdominal obesity, and wealthy nations in 2004. Endocrinology. 2004 Jun;145(6):2633–8. Epub 2004 Mar 24. Review.
- Drapeau V, Therrien F, Richard D, Tremblay A. Is visceral obesity a physiological adaptation to stress? Panminerva Med. 2003 Sep;45(3):189–95. Review.
- Epel ES, McEwen B, Seeman T, Matthews K, Castellazzo G, Brownell KD, Bell J, Ickovics JR. Stress and body shape: stress-induced cortisol secretion is consistently greater among women with central fat. Psychosom Med. 2000 Sep-Oct;62(5):623–32.
- McArdle WD, Katch FI, Katch VL. Exercise Physiology: Energy, Nutrition and Human Performance (2nd edition). Philadelphia: Lea & Febiger, 1986.
- Mokdad AH, Marks JS, Stroup DF, Gerberding JL. Actual causes of death in the United States, 2000. JAMA. 2004 Mar 10;291(10):1238–45. Review.
- President's Council on Physical Fitness and Sports (PCPFS). Accessed online June 20, 2005 at http://fitness.gov/physical_activity_fact_sheet.html

- Ryan N. Physical Fitness–The Active Life–The Nolan Ryan Fitness Guide. Accessed online June 20, 2005 at www.fitness.gov/activelife/nolanryan/ nolanryan.html
- Seckl JR, Morton NM, Chapman KE, Walker BR. Glucocorticoids and 11beta-hydroxysteroid dehydrogenase in adipose tissue. Recent Prog Horm Res. 2004;59:359–93. Review.
- Williams MH. Nutrition for Fitness and Sport. Dubuque: William C. Brown Company Publishers, 1983.

CHAPTER 8: IMPORTANT TIPS TO REMEMBER ON
THE 14-DAY PERRICONE WEIGHT-LOSS DIET

- De Carvalho Papa P, Vargas AM, da Silva JL, Nunes MT, Machado UF. GLUT4 protein is differently modulated during development of obesity in monosodium glutamate-treated mice. Life Sci. 2002 Sep 6;71(16):1917–28.
- De Mello MA, de Souza CT, Braga LR, dos Santos JW, Ribeiro IA, Gobatto CA. Glucose tolerance and insulin action in monosodium glutamate (MSG) obese exercise-trained rats. Physiol Chem Phys Med NMR. 2001;33(1):63–71.
- De Souza CT, Nunes WM, Gobatto CA, de Mello MA. Insulin secretion in monosodium glutamate (MSG) obese rats submitted to aerobic exercise training. Physiol Chem Phys Med NMR. 2003;35(1):43–53.
- Diniz YS, Faine LA, Galhardi CM, Rodrigues HG, Ebaid GX, Burneiko RC, Cicogna AC, Novelli EL. Monosodium glutamate in standard and high-fiber diets: metabolic syndrome and oxidative stress in rats. Nutrition. 2005 Jun;21(6):749–55.
- Franz MJ. Protein: metabolism and effect on blood glucose levels. Diabetes Educ. 1997 Nov-Dec;23(6):643–6, 648, 650–1. Review.
- Geuns JM. Stevioside. Phytochemistry. 2003 Nov;64(5):913–21. Review.
- Hermanussen M, Tresguerres JA. Does high glutamate intake cause obesity? J Pediatr Endocrinol Metab. 2003 Sep;16(7):965–8.
- Keen CL, Holt RR, Oteiza PI, Fraga CG, Schmitz HH. Cocoa antioxidants and cardiovascular health. Am J Clin Nutr. 2005 Jan;81(1 Suppl):298S-303S. Review.
- Layman DK, Baum JI. Dietary protein impact on glycemic control during weight loss. J Nutr. 2004 Apr;134(4):968S-73S. Review.

◆ Lee KW, Kim YJ, Lee HJ, Lee CY. Cocoa has more phenolic phytochemicals and a higher antioxidant capacity than teas and red wine. J Agric Food Chem. 2003 Dec 3;51(25):7292–5.

◆ Pearson DA, Holt RR, Rein D, Paglieroni T, Schmitz HH, Keen CL. Flavanols and platelet reactivity. Clin Dev Immunol. 2005 Mar;12(1):1–9. Review.

◆ Rencuzogullari E, Tuylu BA, Topaktas M, Ila HB, Kayraldiz A, Arslan M, Diler SB. Genotoxicity of aspartame. Drug Chem Toxicol. 2004 Aug;27(3):257–68.

◆ Sasai A. Speech on promoting the spread of chocolate and cocoa in Japan: Programs and results. ICCO, 10 March 1997. The 2nd international symposium of chocolate and cocoa nutrition. Chocolate and Cocoa Association of Japan, 1996.

◆ Sekihashi K, Saitoh H, Sasaki Y. [Genotoxicity studies of stevia extract and steviol by the comet assay]. J Toxicol Sci. 2002 Dec;27 Suppl 1:1–8. Japanese.

◆ Sies H, Schewe T, Heiss C, Kelm M. Cocoa polyphenols and inflammatory mediators. Am J Clin Nutr. 2005 Jan;81(1 Suppl):304S-312S. Review.

◆ Stoclet JC, Chataigneau T, Ndiaye M, Oak MH, El Bedoui J, Chataigneau M, Schini-Kerth VB. Vascular protection by dietary polyphenols. Eur J Pharmacol. 2004 Oct 1;500(1–3):299–313. Review.

◆ Yasukawa K, Kitanaka S, Seo S. Inhibitory effect of stevioside on tumor promotion by 12-O-tetradecanoylphorbol-13-acetate in two-stage carcinogenesis in mouse skin. Biol Pharm Bull. 2002 Nov;25(11):1488–90.

Index

cyanidin, in açaí, 58
cytokines, 19

D

Dadhaniya, Navinchandra, 19
daikon radish sprouts, 145
dairy foods. *See also specific dairy foods*
  beneficial effects of calcium, 77–78
  choose organic brands, 143
  compounds in milk that promote weight-loss branched-chain amino acids, 78
  whey protein, 78
  low-fat probiotic with calcium, 77–81
  soymilk, soy beverages, 224–225
day-by-day diet plan, 164–181
depression, salmon as treatment for, 6
DHA (docosahexaenoic acid), 36, 37
diabetes
  beneficial effects of
    avocados in the diet, 56–57
    fenugreek in the diet, 64
    flaxseeds, 72
    olive oil in the diet, 60
  incidence of, 26
  relation to chronic inflammation, 10
  risk for
    being overweight, 21–22
    insulin resistance, 22
dietary trends, since 1960, 4
diseases and conditions related to chronic inflammation, 10
DMAE (dimethylaminoethanol), 25, 114–115
  dosage recommendations, 115
  in fish, 142
  sources of, 45
  tips, 114

E

Ecco Bello chocolate bar, 149
ECGC, in tea, 133
edamame, 222
Edamame Guacamole, 195

eggplant
  puree, 185
  salad, 189
eggs, from cage-free chickens, 143
Egyptian Chicken Salad, 196
eicosapentaenoic acid (EPA), 36, 37
Elkman, Paul, 130
endocrine organ, areas of fat storage as, 20–21
Environmental Protection Agency (EPA)
  Fish Advisory website, 231
  mercury in fish and shellfish, 229–232
enzymes
  in raw foods, 143–144
  in sprouts, 144
EPA (eicosapentaenoic acid), 36, 37
epinephrine, 127
erythritol, 153
essential fatty acids, 35, 37, 69. *See also* omega-3 essential fatty acids
etouffée, three-fish, with baby artichokes and spicy tomato broth, 216
European Food Information Council (EUFIC) website, 240
European Union, 3
  on growth hormones in beef, 46
exercise, 116–136
  aerobic, 119
  anti-inflammatory benefits of, 116–117
  anti-inflammatory remedies, 136
  energy expenditure chart, 121–122
  health effects of, 121
  how much, how often, 117, 119–121, 124–125
  overexercising, 117
  physical activity fact sheet, 120–121
  resources for, 239
  strength and resistance training, 123–126
    categories of exercises, 123
    how much, how often, 124–125

progressing, 126
  safety tips, 125–126
  stress, stress-related weight gain, and obesity, 127–136
    the cholesterol component, 129–130
    cortisol, the stress/death hormone, 127–128
    how stress promotes weight gain, 128–129
    stress-reducing activities, 130–136
  stretching: reach for flexibility, 122–123
  target heart rate, 120
  tips to get started and keep going, 126–127
  ways to ensure that you exercise regularly, 118–119

F

fagopyritols, 84
Fast Food Nation, 4
fat burning foods, 65–68
  functional weight control factors: anti-inflammatory antioxidants, fiber, phytonutrients, 65
  runners-up: red pepper or crushed red pepper flakes, 67
  top choice: chili peppers and hot chili sauce, 65–66
fats. *See also* specific fats
  in fruits to fight body fat, 55–61
  good fats, 6, 25–26, 146
  recommended, 158
Fats of Life and PUFA newsletter, 239
fenugreek, 64
fiber, 113
  in apples, 49
  in avocados, 55
  in barley, 87
  in beans, 74
  benefits, 145
  in buckwheat, 85
  content of apples, 49
  in flaxseed, 72
  in fruits, 48, 49
  in pears, 51
  recommended intake per day, 145

About the Author

NICHOLAS PERRICONE, M.D., F.A.C.N., is the author of three # 1 *New York Times* best-sellers, *The Perricone Promise, The Perricone Prescription,* and *The Wrinkle Cure,* as well as *The Clear Skin Prescription.*

Dr. Perricone is a board-certified clinical and research dermatologist, and adjunct professor of medicine at the Michigan State University's College of Human Medicine. He is certified by the American Board of Dermatology, is a fellow of the New York Academy of Sciences, and a fellow of the American College of Nutrition. He is also a fellow of the American Academy of Dermatology and the Society of Investigative Dermatology. Dr. Perricone has served as assistant clinical professor of dermatology at Yale School of Medicine and as chief of dermatology at the state of Connecticut's Veterans Hospital. He is regarded as the father of the Inflammation Theory of Aging.

As an internationally renowned research scientist and inventor, Dr. Perricone is the recipient of the Eli Whitney Award for his significant contributions to science, invention, and technology. He holds dozens of U.S. and international patents for the treatment of skin and systemic disease, and for the use of topical anti-inflammatories for reversing and preventing damage to skin caused by factors such as age, the sun, the environment, and hormonal changes.

Dr. Perricone is also the creator and host of a series of award-winning public television specials airing nationally on PBS. He is a popular guest on national television, appearing on the *Today* show, *20/20, Larry King, Good Morning America, The View,* CNN, Fox, *Extra, Access Hollywood,* as well as many news broadcasts. He has been featured in the *New York Times, The Wall Street Journal, Vogue, Harper's Bazaar, W, Forbes, People,* and *USA Today.*

Visit the author's website at www.nvperriconemd.com.

About the Type

This book was set in Baskerville, a typeface which was designed by John Baskerville, an amateur printer and type founder, and cut for him by John Handy in 1750. The type became popular again when The Lanston Monotype Corporation of London revived the classic Roman face in 1923. The Mergenthaler Linotype Company in England and the United States cut a version of Baskerville in 1931, making it one of the most widely used typefaces today.